X 3527
All rights reserved
This 1994 edition published by Grange Books
An imprint of Grange Books PLC
The Grange, Grange Yard, London SE1 3AG

© *1994 Loveline Publishing*

CONCEIVED BY *Waterbridge Books*
DESIGNED BY *Chris Humour*
EDITED BY *Virginia Comfrey*
TYPESET BY *Chris Lanaway*
Photographs © *Loveline Publishing*

Printed and bound in Italy

ISBN 1-85627-493-4

THE *Lovers'* *Guide* TO
KAMA SUTRA

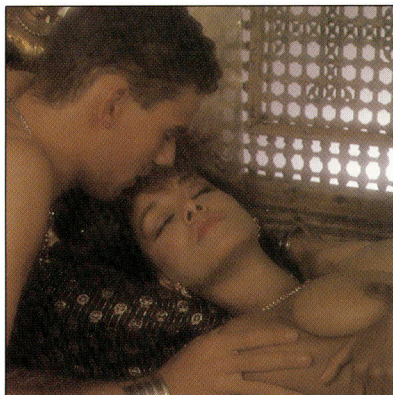

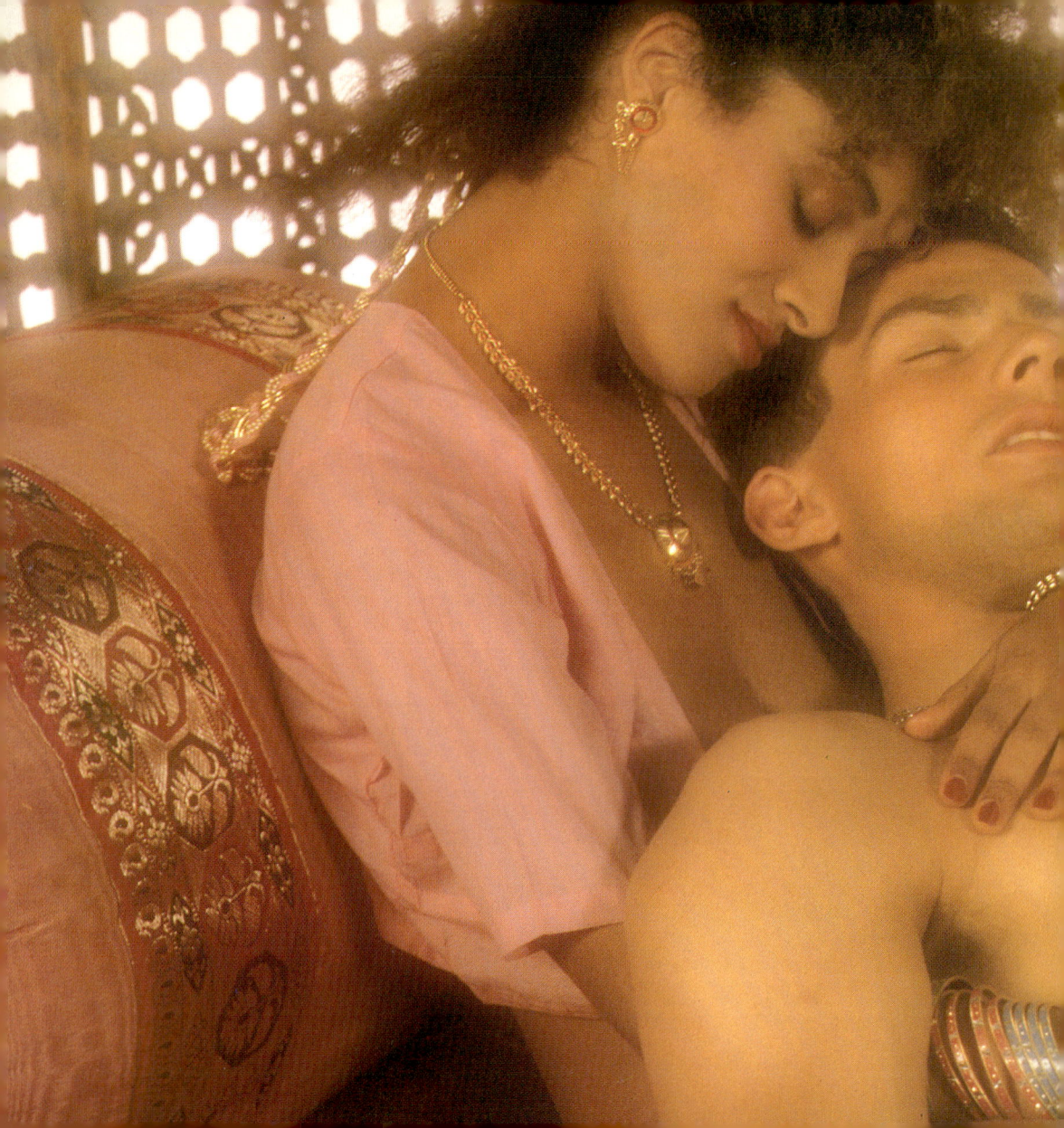

THE *Lovers'* *Guide* TO
KAMA SUTRA

Grange
BOOKS

The Kama Sutra *is probably the most famous sex manual in the world. Although there are dozens of others available, this ancient document retains its remarkable power to excite and enthrall new readers.*

At the very heart of the Kama Sutra *lies the notion that sex is one of life's joys and that it is actually a part of everyday living, to be spoken, sung, danced and thought about; to be discussed openly and taught as a skill with reading, writing and conversation.*

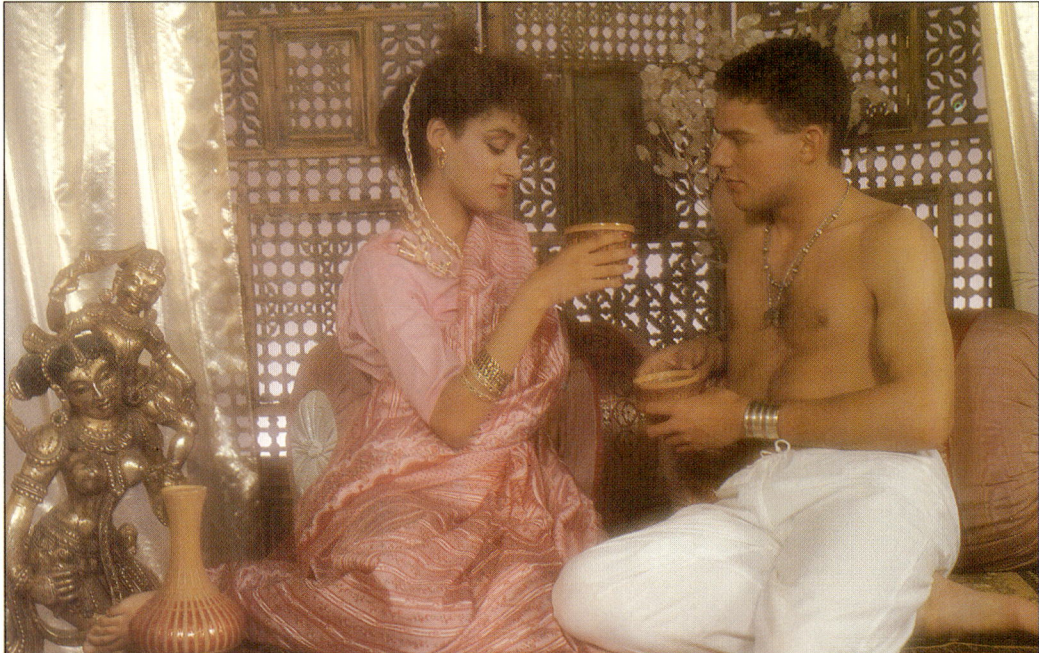

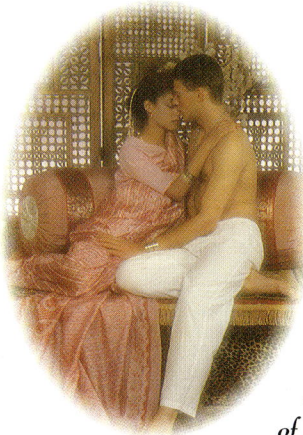

Apart from its famous descriptions of positions for sexual intercourse, the Kama Sutra also contains a considerable amount of related sexual information.

Erection creams, delay sprays, sex aids, sex toys and aphrodisiacs are not the inventions of a degenerate twentieth century. The Kama Sutra provides information about all of these things, as well as informative notes on the way to conduct long-term relationships.

The title Kama Sutra is generally translated as 'Aphorisms of Love', or sometimes rather more romantically as 'Songs of Love' or even 'Love's Melodies'. In Hindu mythology, Vishnu was the 'Lord of the Universe', known as 'the Preserver' and as 'Lord of the Waters'. He was also said to be the ruler of man's erotic impulses and desires. His consort was Lakshmi - 'beautiful as ten million rising suns' - and also regarded as the embodiment of sensuality.

Their son was Kama - the god of love. He was blessed with eternal youth and great beauty. Many writers have remarked on his resemblance to Cupid, since Kama also shoots arrows of flowers from a bow. He rides on a dove and is particularly associated with springtime. Kama was believed to hover, invisibly, over all acts of love. His wife was Rati, regarded as the embodiment of sensual love.

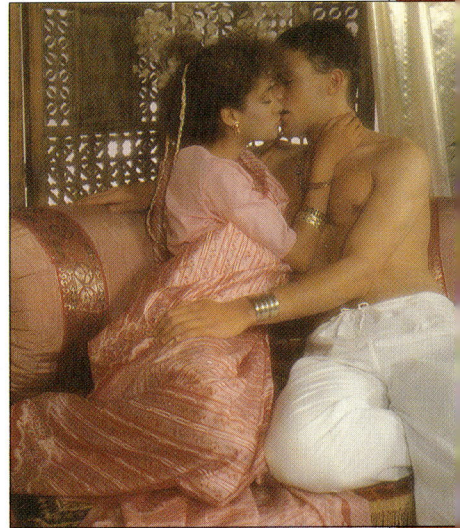

Kissing is the second 'art of love' described in the *Kama Sutra*.

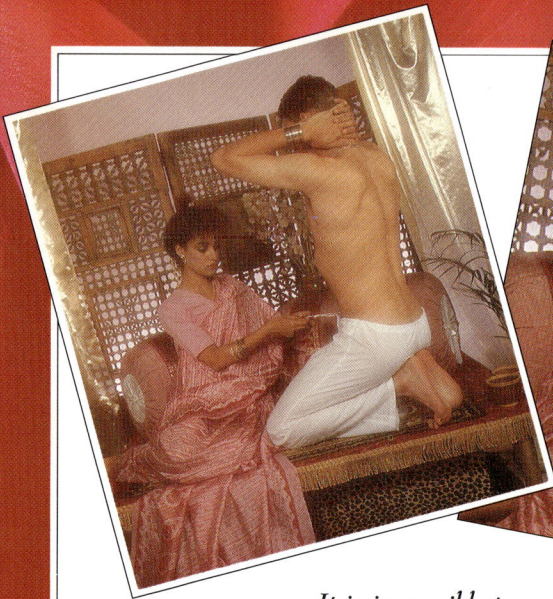

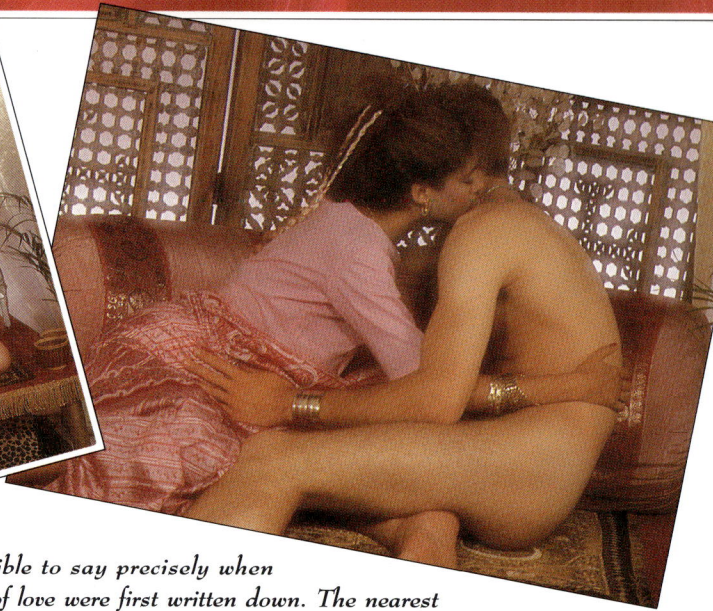

It is impossible to say precisely when Kama's songs of love were first written down. The nearest Sanskrit scholars can get is to place the work somewhere between the first and fourth centuries A.D. Its author is always referred to as Vatsyayana as he belonged to the Vatsyayana sect.

The first English translation of the Kama Sutra was made by the charismatic and eminent Orientalist and explorer, Sir Richard Burton. It was the result of comparing copies from the libraries of Bombay, Benares, Calcutta and Jaipur and was printed in 1883.

The Kama Sutra has been translated several times since - and today ranks as one of the great classics of erotic literature.

This Guide offers a resumé of the Kama Sutra, emphasising those sections on sexual techniques most interesting to modern Western readers. The photographs accompanying the text have been designed to recreate in modern terms the sexual advice given in the Kama Sutra.

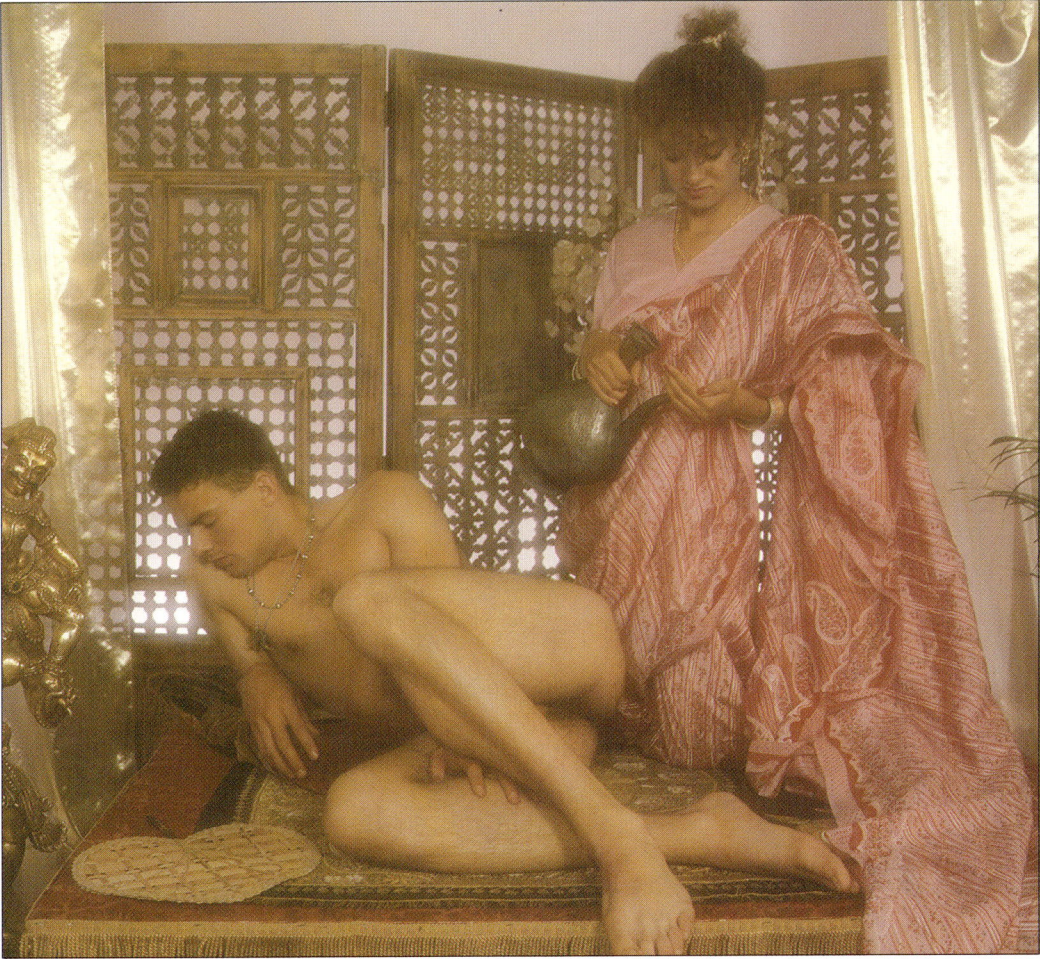

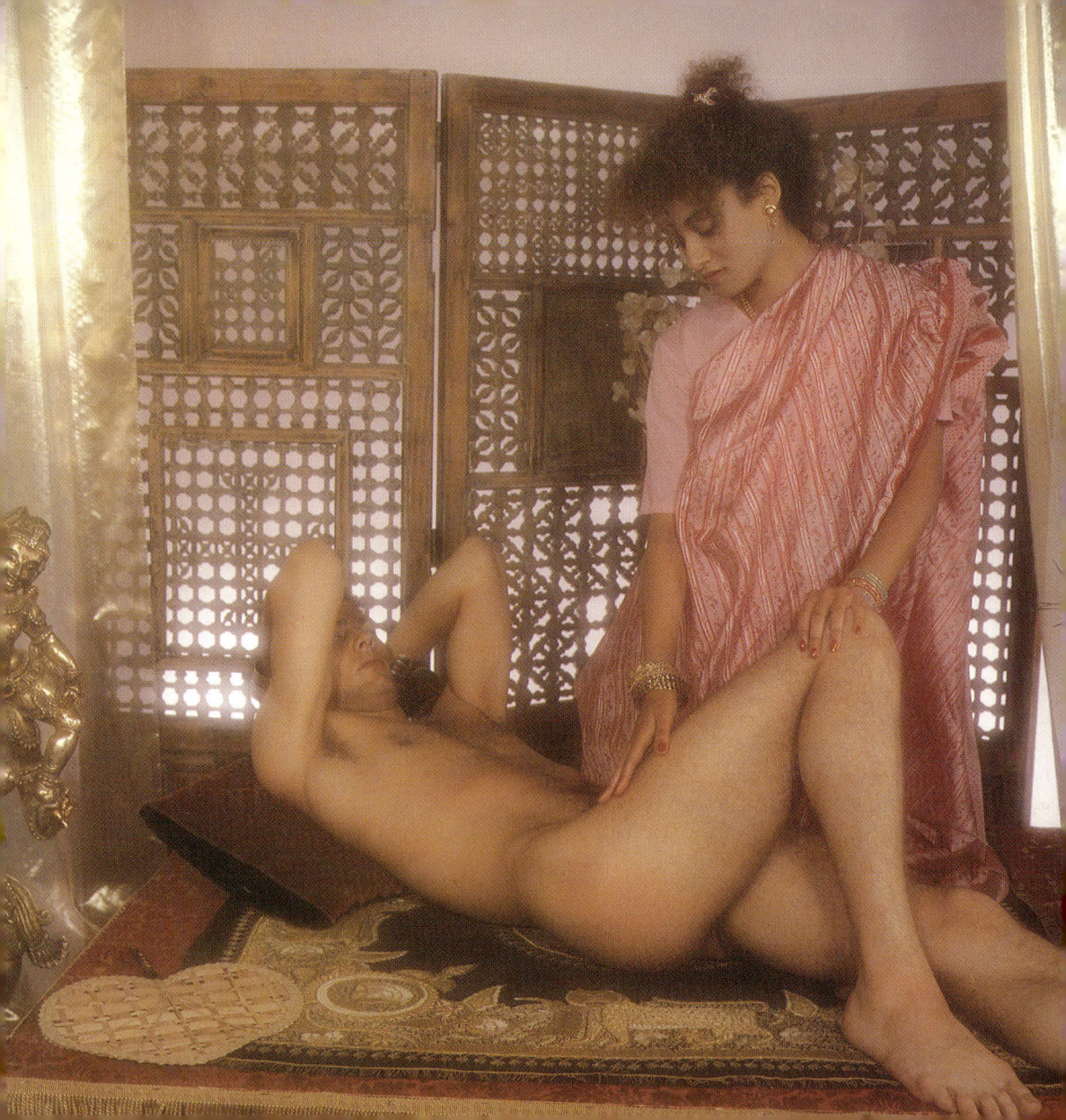

An Erotic Lifestyle

Anybody picking up the Kama Sutra and expecting a highly-charged 'pornographic' read is bound to be disappointed. The section which deals with sexual union is substantial, detailed and explicit and, when read carefully, is extremely erotic. But this is only one section of a fairly long treatise. Vatsyayana is, in fact, dealing with the whole area of love, relationships, lifestyle, and the proper conduct of his readers.

However, all this other material is pervaded with an acute sexual and sensual awareness which can be best appreciated if one understands a little of the Hindu attitude to the good life, and to sex in particular. To the Hindu, the good, or complete, life meant that the individual must attempt to achieve harmony between three essential activities. These are Dharma, which means a life of religious obligation; Artha, which refers to economic and political activity, and Kama, which is the life of the senses. The Hindu philosophy recognised the importance of all three strands but insisted they should be studied and practised equally so that an appropriate blend of all three was achieved.

The concept of sex as an art form, and one that should be studied as much by women as by men, is one of the most powerful themes of the Kama Sutra, and related to this is the attitude it reveals towards women. Hindu society at the time was highly organised and well-regulated, but within these rules women enjoyed an amount of freedom and autonomy. It was considered acceptable for young women to study the Kama Sutra and,

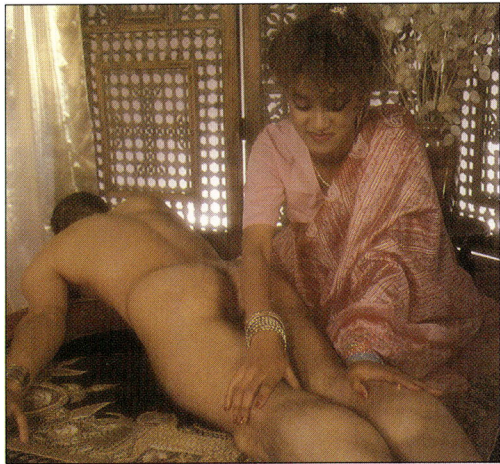

Massage and oiling of the body is described as 'shampooing' by Vatsyayana. He does not class it as an embrace 'because it is performed at a different time, for a different reason and has a different character'.

If the woman is a virgin, the man is advised to approach gently, paying attention to her breasts first, undressing her. . .

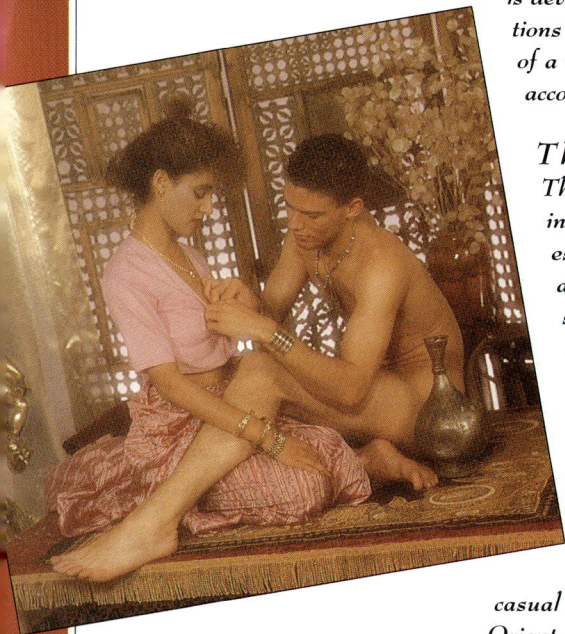

although marriages were arranged, or negotiated, Vatsyayana believed in love and makes the point that unless a young couple are together a lot and share entertainments, games and social activities, then love cannot begin to blossom. Quite a lot of space is devoted to the importance of courtship and - in the sex instructions (to be considered in detail later) - to the gradual arousing of a virgin, or newly-married girl, from shyness or fear to an accomplished and eager partner.

The Secrets of Sex

The section of the Kama Sutra which deals with sexual instruction opens with a short chapter which gets down to the essentials with no preliminaries, in this case the essentials are: genital size (male and female), degree of passion (or sexual excitement) and the time taken for both the man and the woman to reach orgasm.

One aspect of writing and talking openly about sex, which still bothers both professionals as well as the person in the street, is the question of what words to use to describe the all-important organs. Either we use technical/medical terms which tend to seem distant and cold ('penis' and 'vagina'). Or we can try for a colloquial tone and use the slang words most commonly used in casual conversation. The sexual commentators of India and the Orient, however, seemed able to devise many elegant and lovely synonyms for the genitals - clear in meaning and easy to use. Thus, for the penis one can find, according to country, 'The Jade Stalk', 'Yang Pagoda', 'Jade Sceptre', and so on. For the vagina one finds 'Jade Gate', 'Precious Gate', 'Cinnabar Crevice', and 'Open Melon'.

Throughout the Kama Sutra the words used are lingam for the penis and yoni for the vagina. These are the words that will be used throughout this commentary.

The opening of Vatsyayana's section on sex (Kinds of Union) asserts that there are three classes of man, which he calls the hare, the bull and the horse according to the size of their lingam. Similarly, there are three classes of woman, defined according to the depth of their yoni, and these he calls the female deer, the mare and the female elephant.

No measurements are given, but a later sex manual, called the Ananga Ranga, which draws on the Kama Sutra and other books for its information, does suggest that the lingam of the hare is about five inches long, that of the bull is seven inches and that of the horse up to ten inches. The depth of the deer's yoni is about five inches, that of the mare about seven inches and that of the elephant around ten inches. Physical characteristics are deduced from these dimensions, too, so the horse is described as being tall and muscular; the deer woman is soft and youthful and so on. Personality traits and even the scent or taste of genital secretions are also deduced: the hare's semen is sweetish, for example, and the elephant-woman's love juice smells like the secretions of mating elephants.

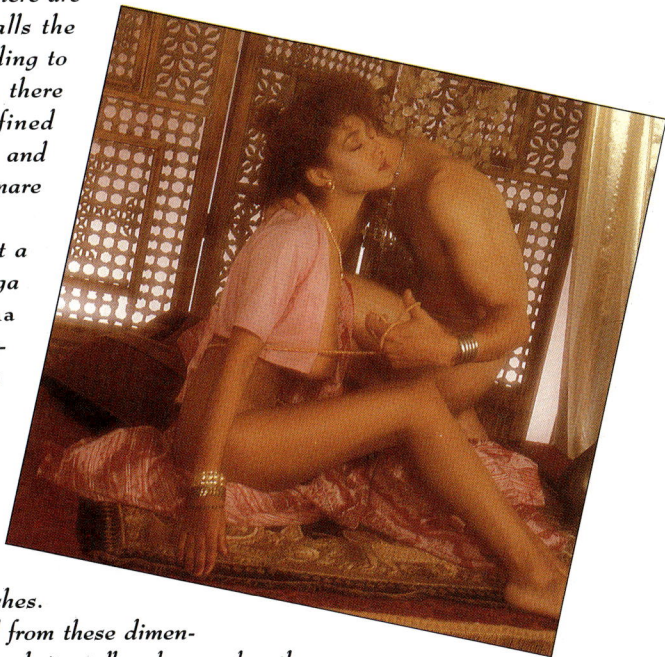

... he should also stroke her hair and take her face between his hands for kissing.

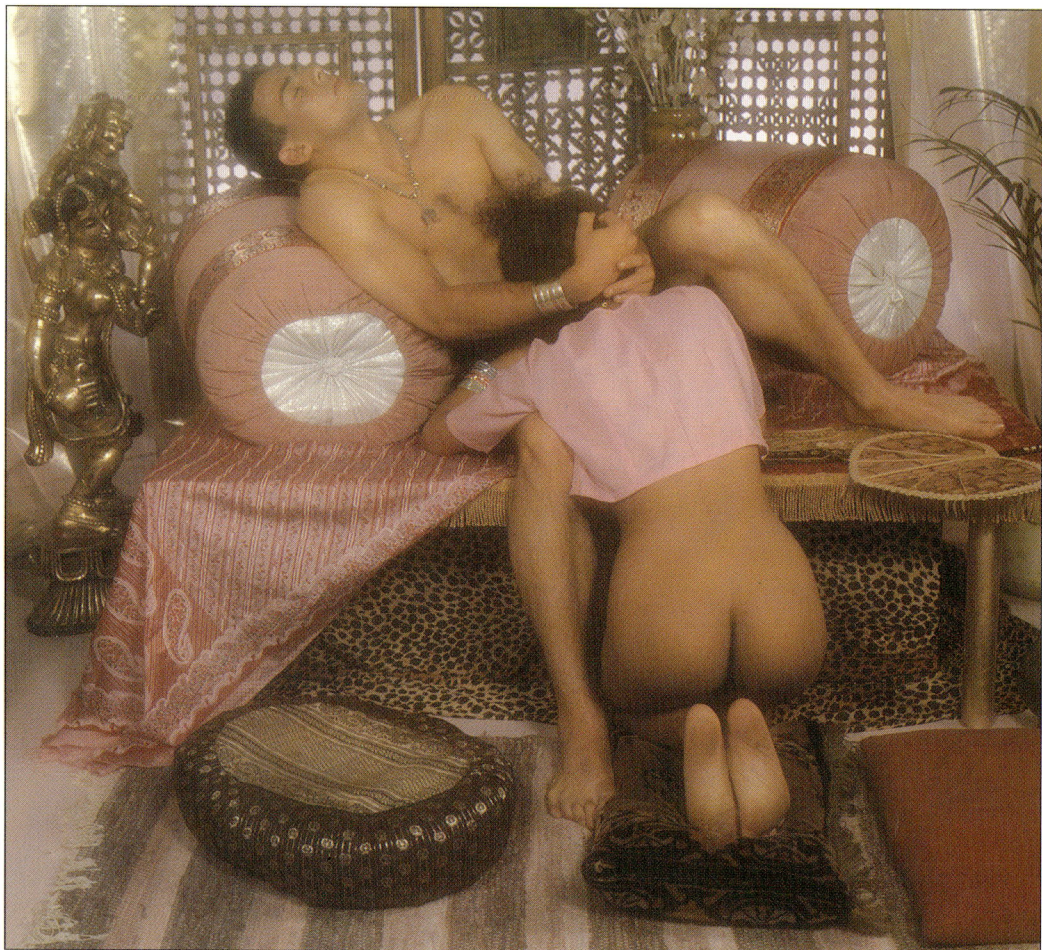

Vatsyayana goes on to enumerate the variations of sexual union possible between the six types of lingam and yoni and defines nine altogether. He states that the 'equal' unions are the most successful - that is hare/deer, bull/mare and horse/elephant. He then divides the six 'mismatches' into sub categories, listing 'high' unions and 'low' unions. High unions are when the male exceeds the female in size; low unions are when the woman exceeds the man in size.

High unions are judged preferable to low unions because with the latter it is difficult to satisfy the female.

This list of ideal and slightly less than ideal couplings provides an introduction and a rationale for the various sexual positions described in such detail later. Many of them are designed so that both partners can get the maximum pleasure out of their union.

The people for whom the Kama Sutra was a major text book did not lead lives of sexual monogamy. Not only might a nagarika (a citizen of culture and leisure) have several wives, he would also enjoy the favours of courtesans now and then. So in the course of a year his lingam might well meet yonis of many sizes and many experiences. The Kama Sutra reminds him to be aware of this and shows him how to prepare for it.

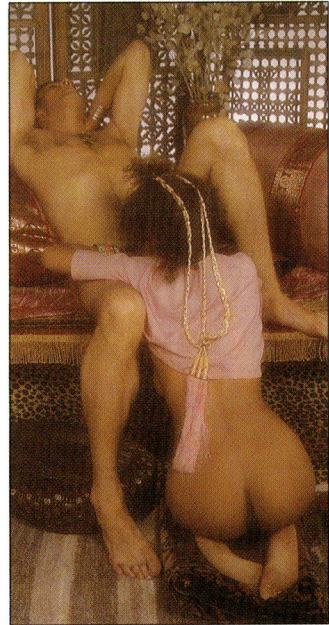

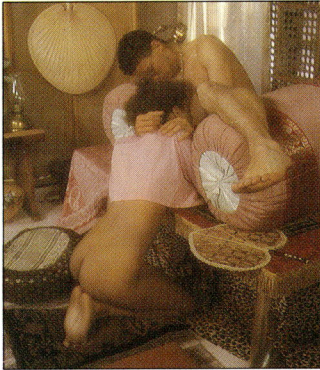

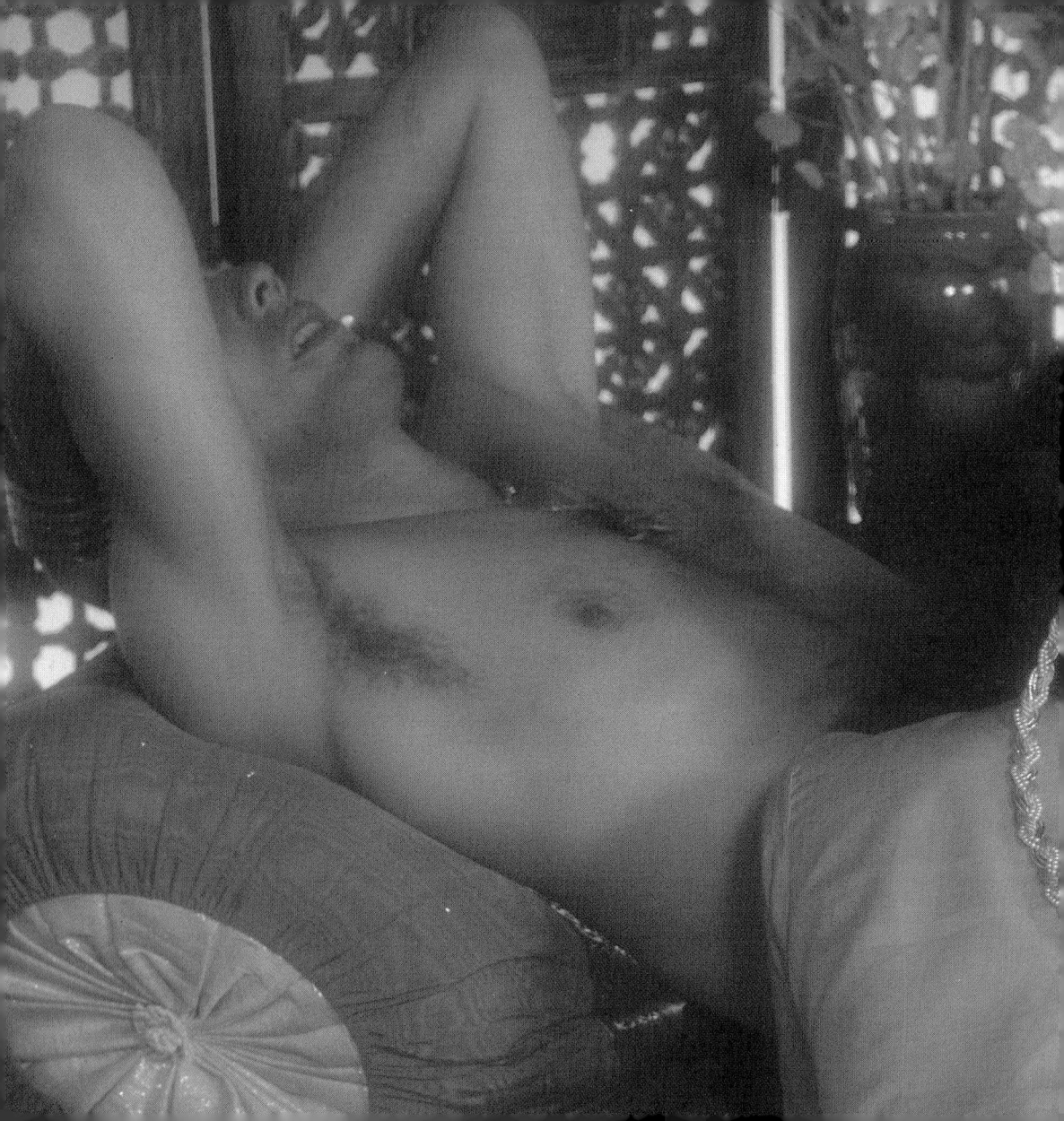

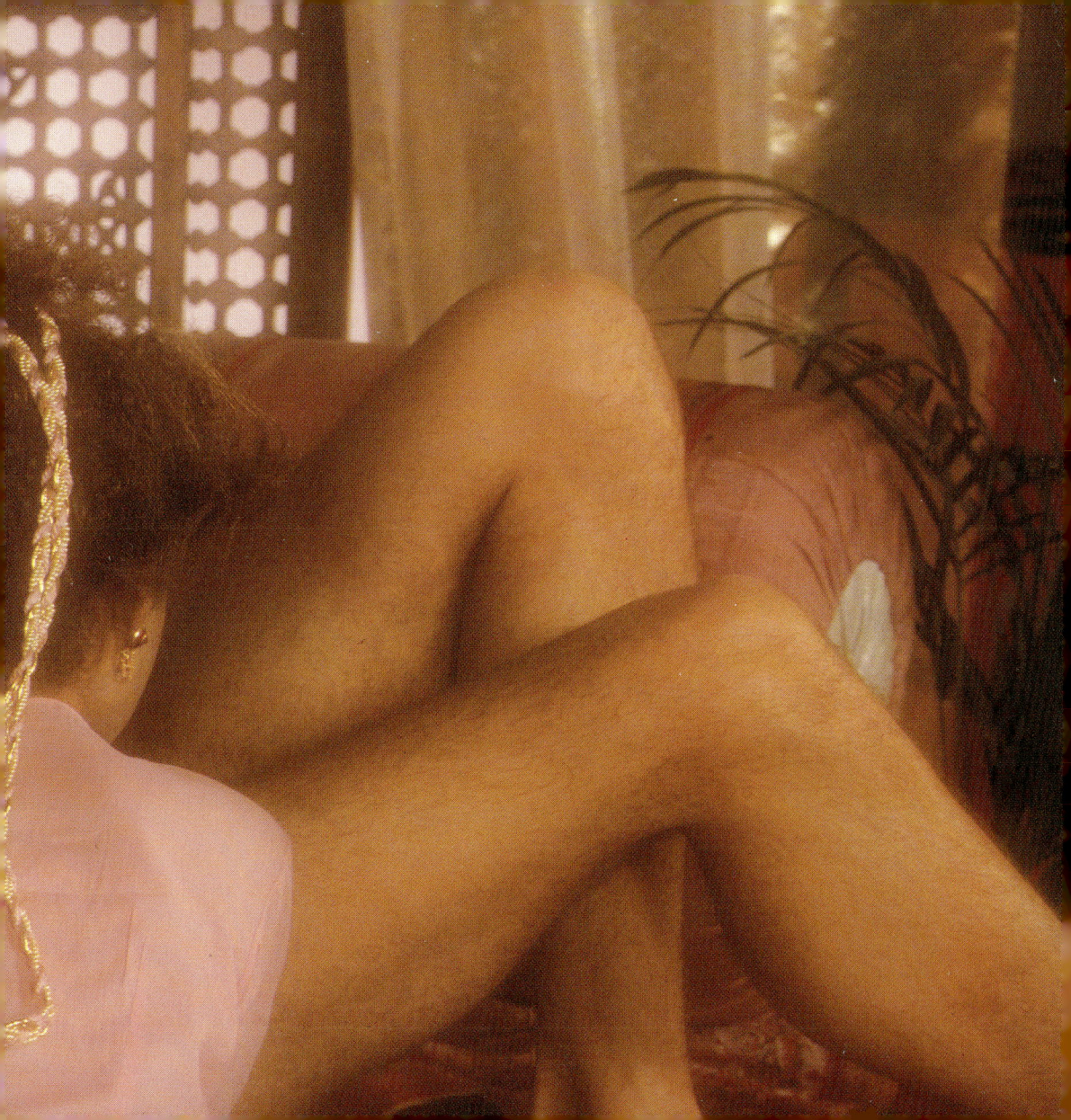

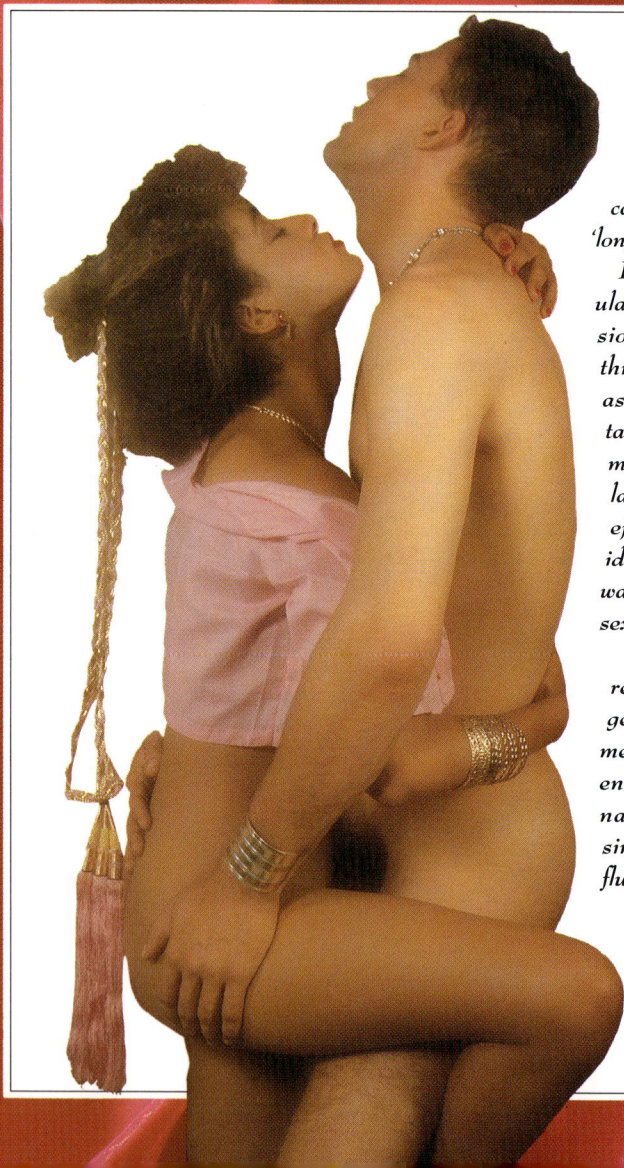

Vatsyayana offers a third group of sexual categories based on the length of time it takes a man or woman to achieve orgasm, which he calls 'short-timed', the 'moderate-timed' and the 'long-timed', which are, of course, self-explanatory.

Linked in with this is the concept of female ejaculation. The Kama Sutra refers to female emission as 'the fall of semen' and seems to equate this phenomenon exactly with male ejaculation - as the manifestation of orgasm (a word, incidentally, not used in the book). So some of the arguments are based on the idea that women ejaculate throughout intercourse, whereas men only ejaculate at their climax; others depend on the idea that women and men ejaculate in the same way and at the same moment in their individual sexual cycles.

Interestingly, the Kama Sutra makes no reference to the physical details of the female genital organs, the inner and outer lips are not mentioned, nor is the clitoris (not even by inference). The sages who were happy to debate the nature of the female orgasm at length quite simply knew that women did enjoy emissions of fluid and these were more intense and more copious when the woman reached the moments of greatest excitement.

The conclusion is that men and women do indeed feel the same kind of sensations and pleasures when making love, but, bearing

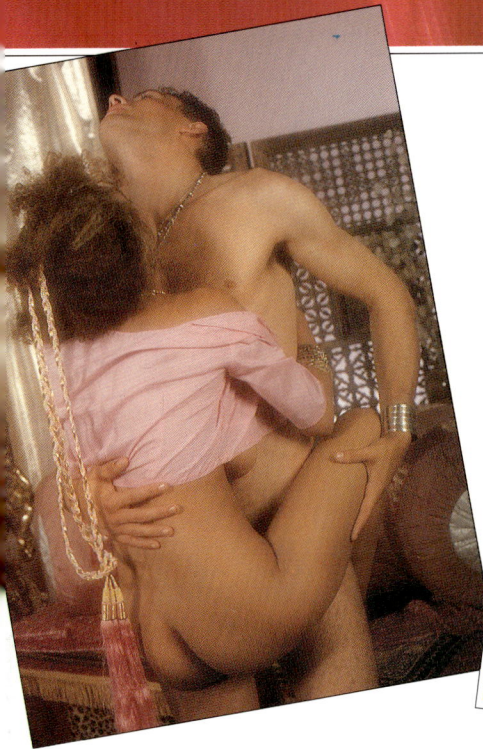

This is the standing embrace known as 'Climbing the Tree', in which the woman clings to the man like a creeper entwining a tree. She is instructed to make little sounds of singing and cooing while doing this.

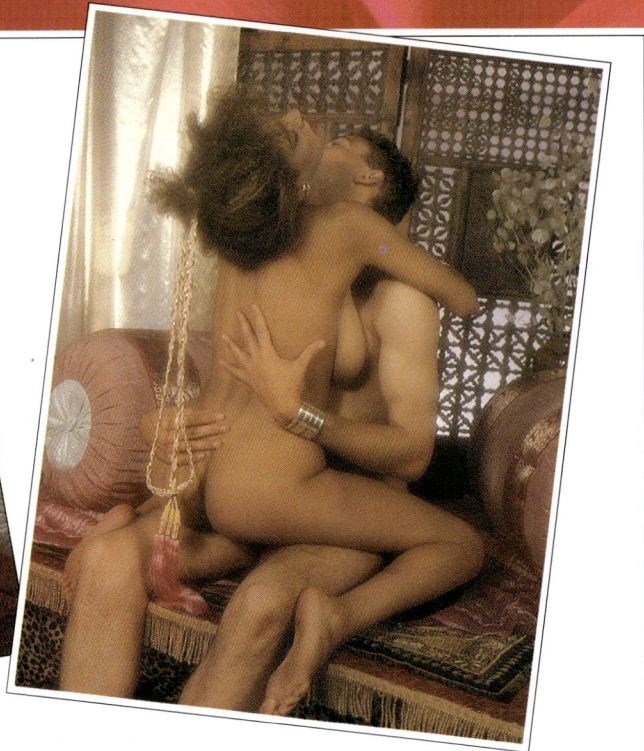

in mind the various permutations of sizes and types possible, in each kind of sexual union it is important that the man should vary his style, approach and technique as seems appropriate.

After this general chapter, there follow more detailed instructions in the art of love.

The arts of love described fall into six sections: embracing, kissing, scratching with the nails, biting, striking and sexual positions. In each category different variations are described with precision and given particular names.

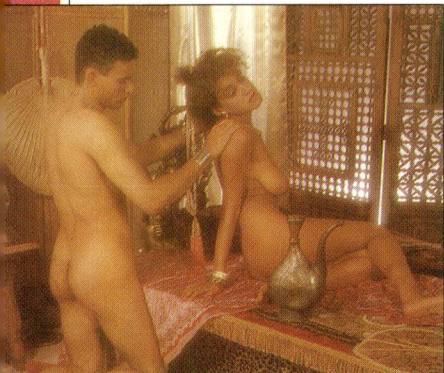

It must be emphasised that all these gestures and positions were not intended, or prescribed, as individual practices but were, rather, expected to feature in the general and increasingly passionate flow of lovemaking. However, as already made clear, for the readers of the Kama Sutra sex and lovemaking were arts to be studied, so all the gestures and kinds of embraces and kisses had their own symbolic significance and examples of them can be found in painting, sculpture and poetry.

The Kama Sutra's first detailed lesson concerns the embrace. In a sense, all contact between the bodies of the two lovers can be termed an embrace and the author emphasises that to him the embrace 'indicates the mutual love of a man and woman who have come together'. But even with this proviso in mind it is clear that an embrace has a wide range of implication, from a casual squeeze of affection to the deeply passionate entwining of limbs.

The first two kinds of embrace described take place only between people who are still getting to know each other and haven't yet quite made their intentions absolutely plain. So they may be regarded as the very first moves in the game of love.

The 'Touching Embrace' is simply when a man makes an excuse to pass close to a woman

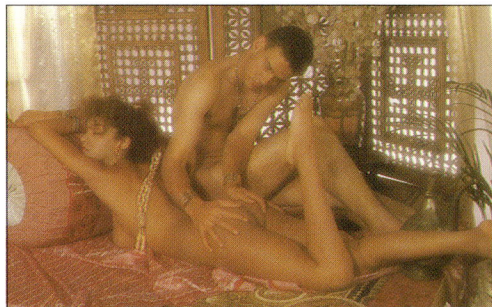

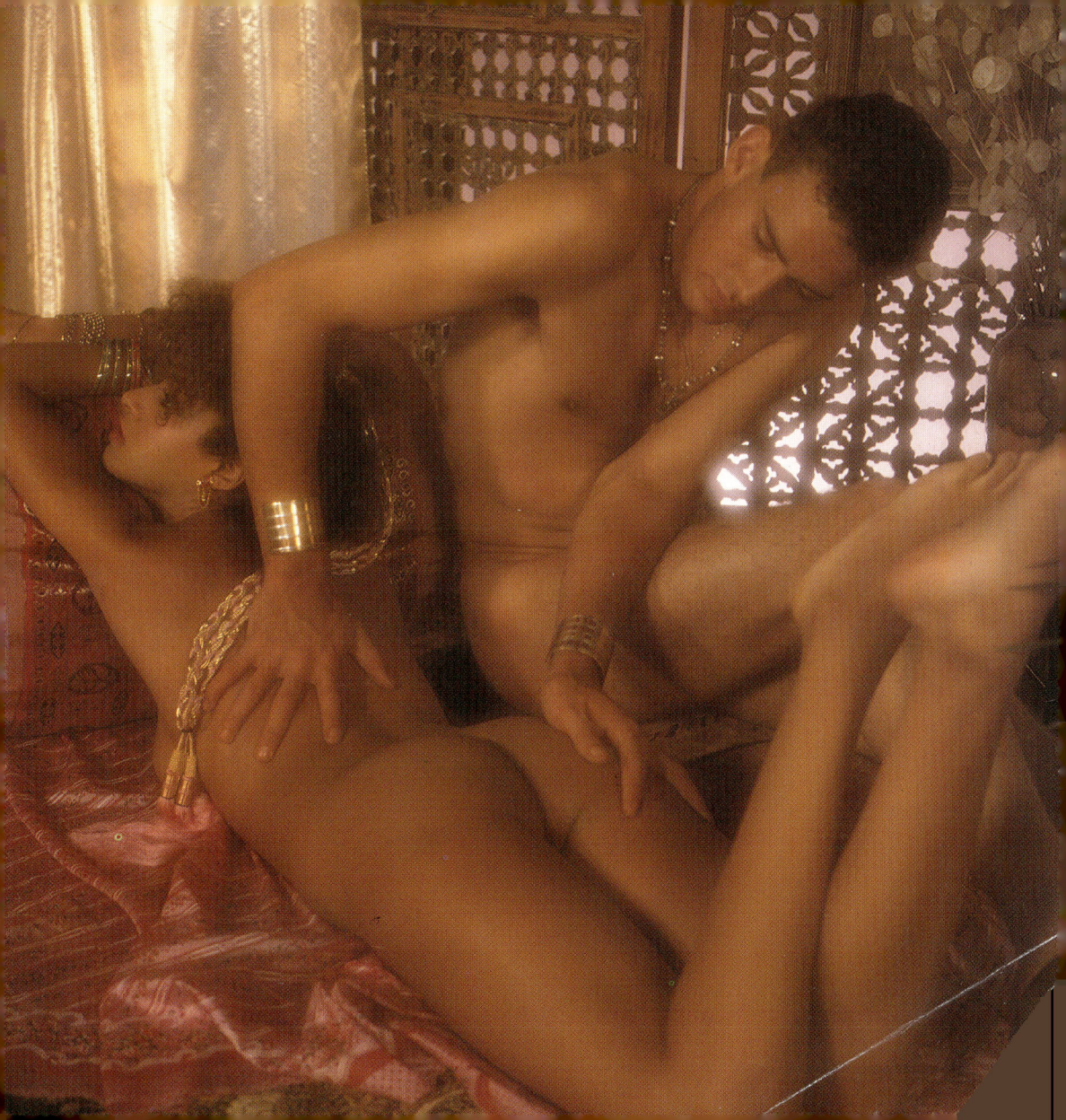

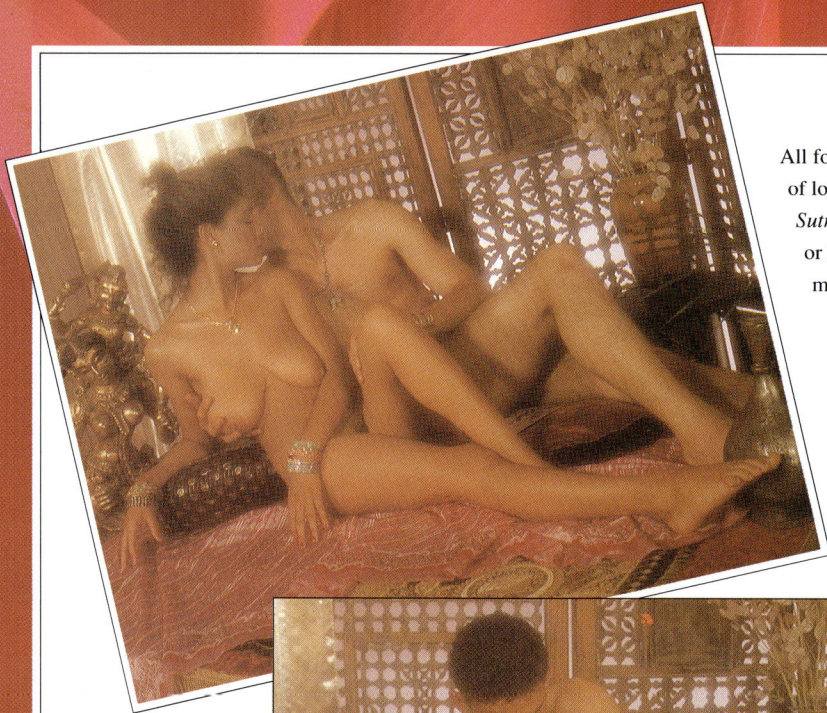

All forms of embracing – 'the second art of love' are sanctioned by the *Kama Sutra* if they help to intensify foreplay or heighten the passion of the moment.

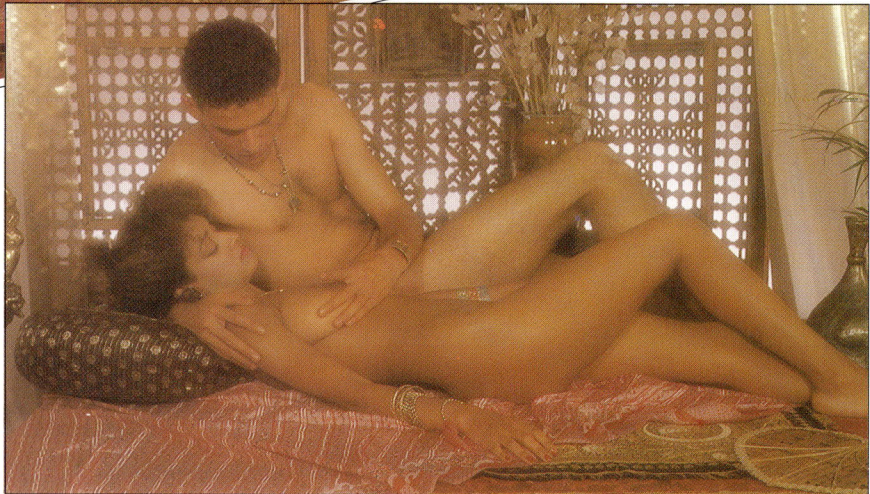

and almost accidentally rubs his body against hers. On one of the moonlit picnics or mixed bathing parties the nagarika who enjoyed such a casual brush could find it electrifying in its implications.

Rather more obvious is the second embrace, called the 'Piercing Embrace'. In this example it is the woman who makes the move. Under some pretext she manages to press her breasts against the man who acknowledges what she has done with a return pressure or even a gentle touch with his hand.

Then, as the couple become more intimate and have made their mutual intentions clear, they can enjoy the 'Rubbing Embrace' which happens as their bodies rub closely against each other as they walk side by side. And when one presses the other's body forcibly up against a wall or pillar and leans on her or him, then this is called a 'Pressing Embrace'. All these four kinds of contact would be acceptable in public places and would perhaps cause a little amusement to the older people as they watched the young couple growing closer in this way.

The next two kinds of embrace belong to lovers who are intimate with each other, and are done in a standing position. First there is 'The Twining of a Creeper', when the woman clings to the man like a beautiful, flowering plant growing around a sturdy tree. She places her hand on the back of his head and bends it down towards her for a kiss and looks lovingly up at him. The other standing embrace pursues the imagery of nature and is called 'The

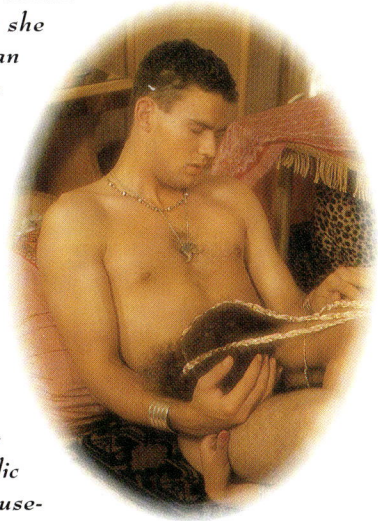

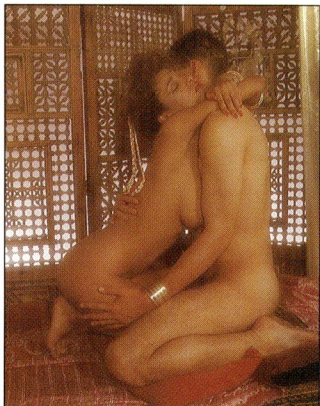

Climbing of a Tree' with the man cast again in the role of tree. She places one of her feet on his and raises her other leg level with his thigh. One of her arms encircles his neck and the other rests on his shoulders as though she were about to climb up his body.

The final pair of formal embraces described are intended to happen at the time of sexual intercourse. The lovers are lying on their bed and they embrace each other so closely and so tightly that the arms and thighs of one are completely encircled by the arms and thighs of the other. This embrace has the name of 'Mixing Sesame Seed and Rice'. 'The Mixture of Milk and Water' is the most passionate of the embraces and demands that the couple entwine passionately, as if they wanted to enter into each other's body. This can be engaged in from a sitting, standing or lying position.

As a kind of footnote, four further embraces are noted, each referring to a particular part of the body. There is the 'Embrace of the Thighs', when one or both of the thighs of a lover are pressed forcibly between the partner's. There is the 'Embrace of the Mid-section' - that is, hips, loins and thighs. There is the 'Embrace of the Breasts', which involves the man asserting his naked chest against the bared breasts of his lover and pressing firmly. This is another embrace which can be enjoyed with one partner sitting on the other's knee. Then there is the particularly

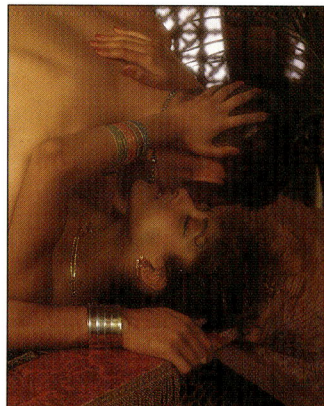

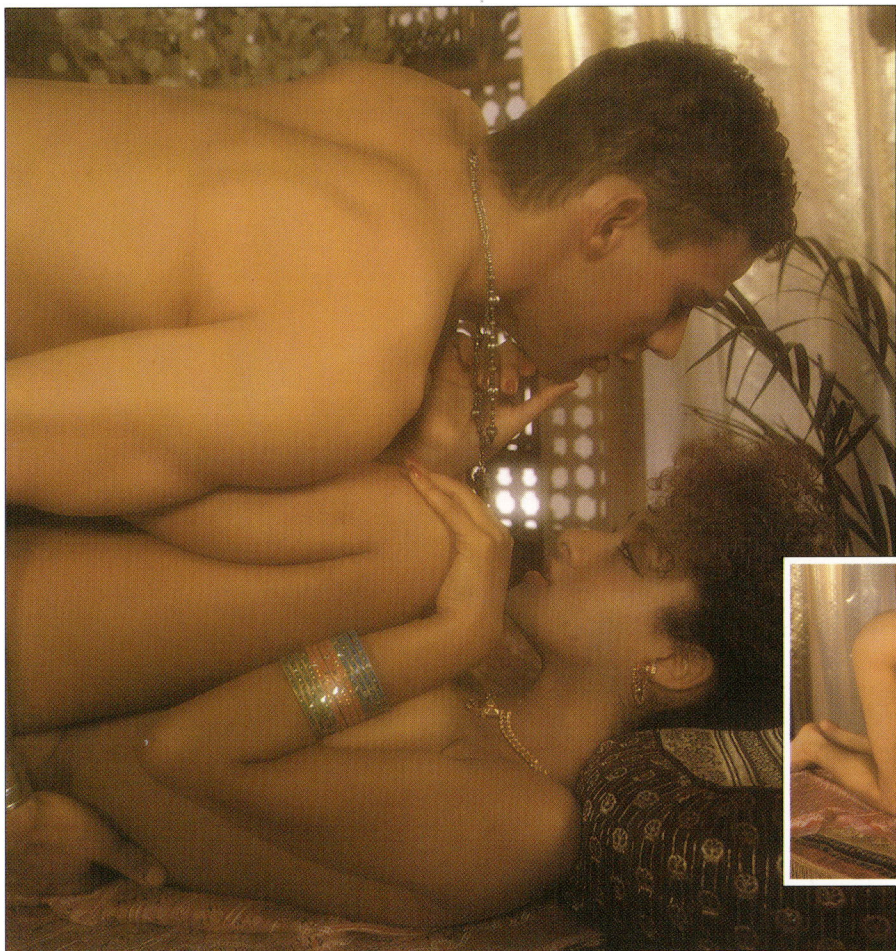

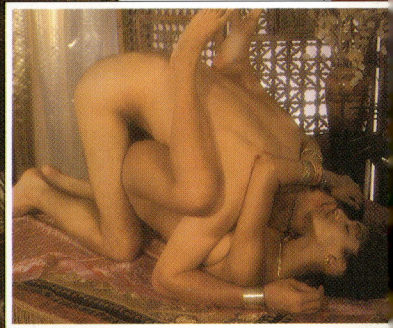

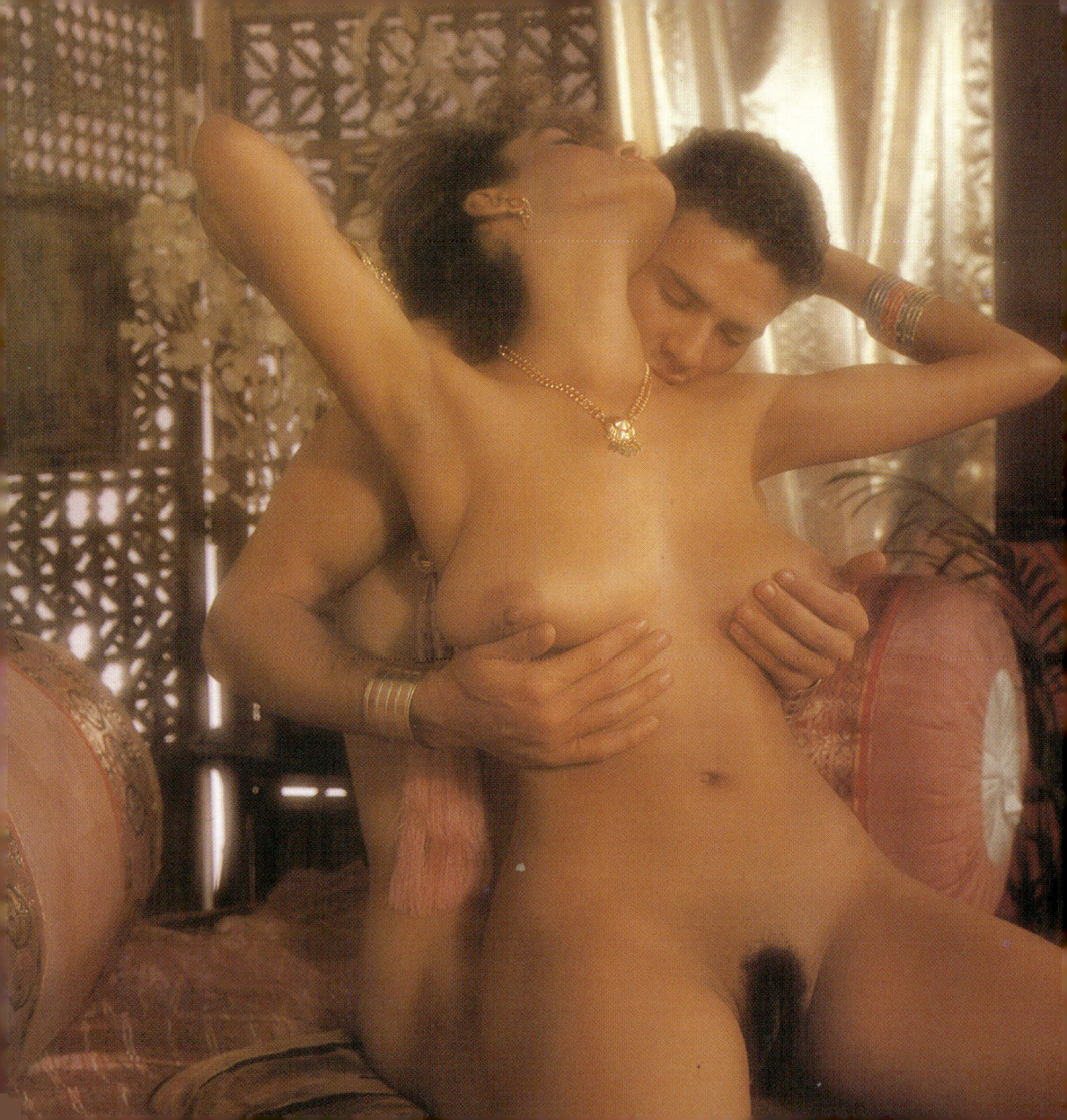

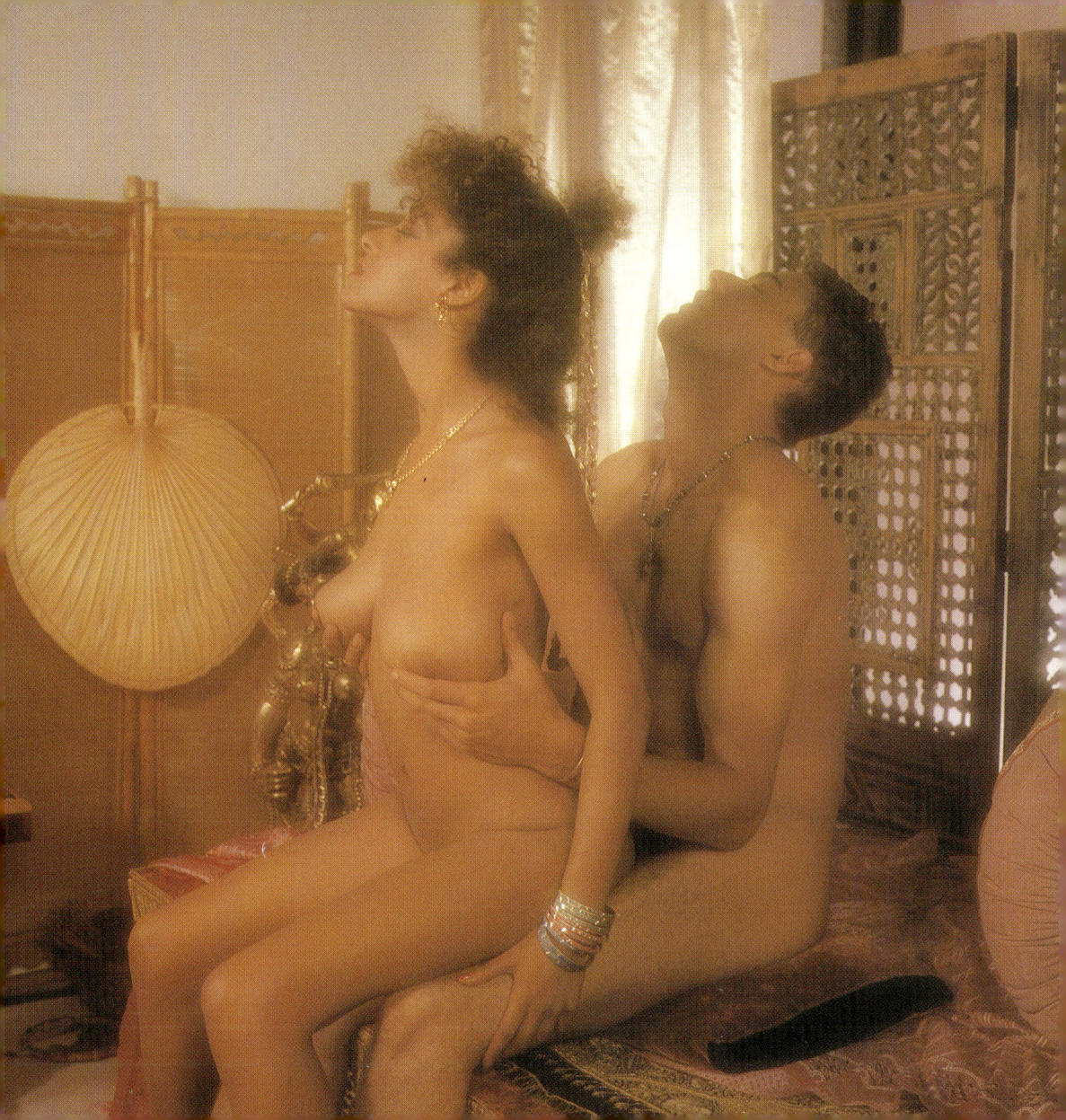

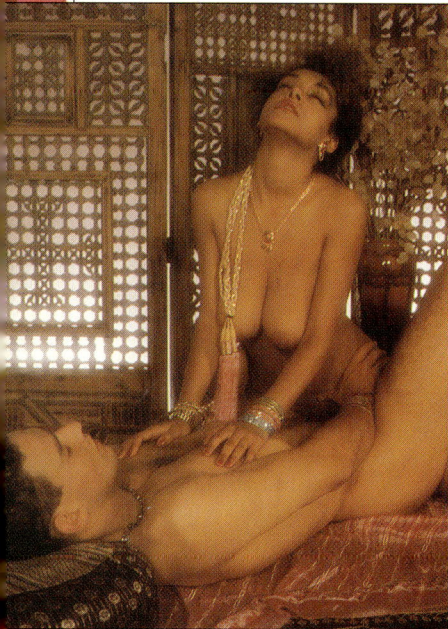

gentle and tender 'Embrace of the Forehead', when either lover touches the other's mouth, eyes and forehead with his or her own.

This short chapter ends on a note of refreshing realism. Actually, any embrace, even if it is not mentioned in the Kama Sutra, is admissible in the cause of sexual enjoyment if it helps to heighten passion.

Before discussing his next subject - kissing - Vatsyayana tries to make it clear that he is not setting out some rigid formula for the correct time and order of foreplay. Anything can be done at any time, he comments, because love ignores set routines. He does feel that when making love for the first time, a couple should kiss in moderation only.

The proper places for kissing include the forehead, the eyes, the cheeks, the throat, the breasts, the lips and inside the mouth. The lower body and the genital regions are not mentioned.

It is, however, the mouth which is of supreme importance, because the coming together of lips, the probing of the tongue and the exchange of body fluids involved in a kiss represent a close approximation to sexual intercourse itself.

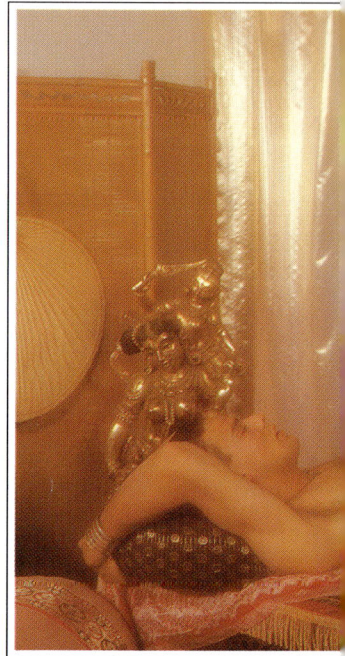

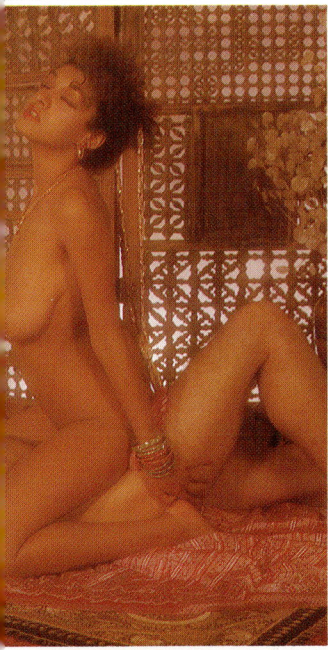

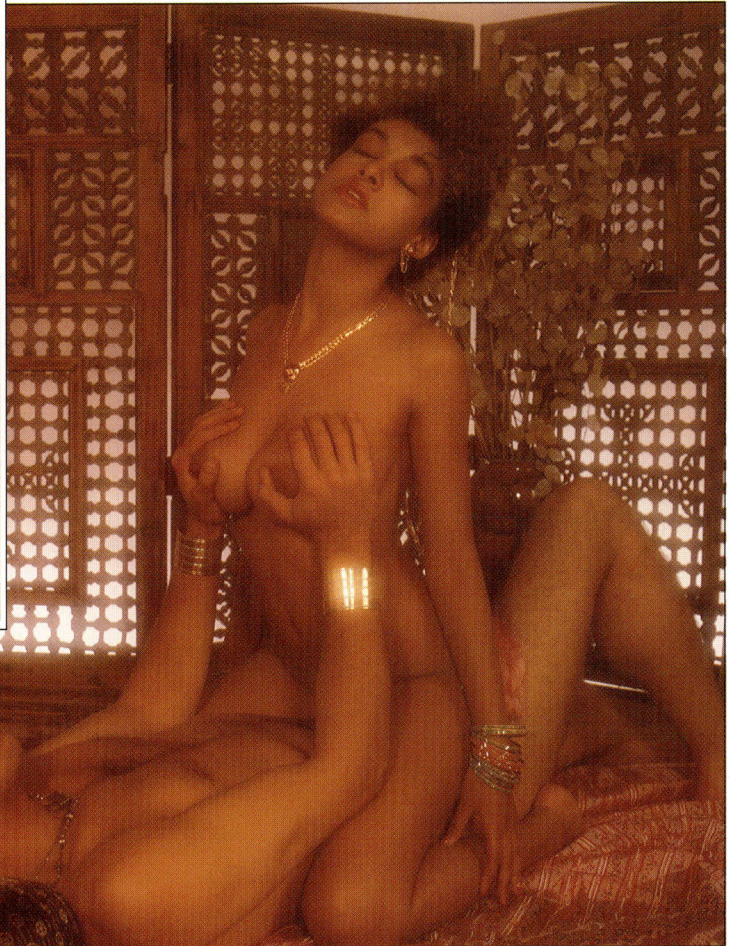

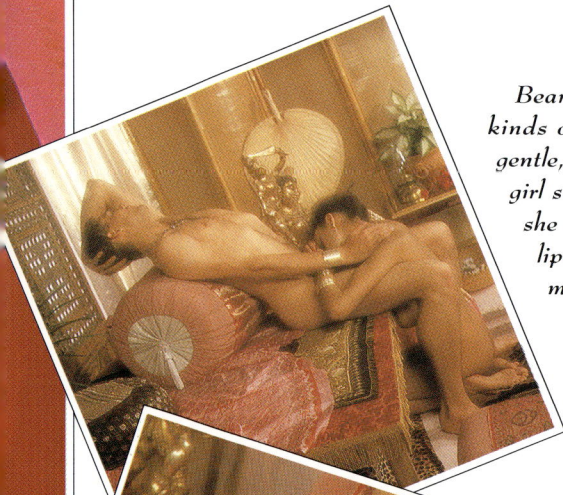

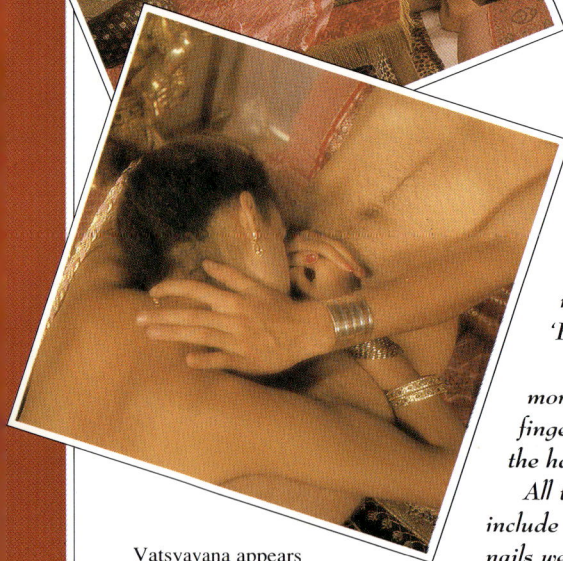

Vatsyayana appears to consider oral sex to be a special form of massage.

Bearing this in mind, the teacher begins by explaining three kinds of kiss most suitable for a young girl. These kisses are gentle, exploratory and tender. The 'Nominal Kiss' is when the girl simply brushes the mouth of her lover with her own. When she is a little more confident she may wish to touch the man's lip when he presses it to her mouth. To this end she should move her lower lip only, not the upper one. This is the 'Throbbing Kiss'. Thirdly, she can touch her lover's lip with her tongue while, at the same time, holding his hands.

Other kisses are listed according to the position of the faces and the amount of pressure used. Interesting is what is known as the 'Greatly Pressed Kiss', which requires the lower lips to be held between two fingers, touched with the tongue and then pressed strongly. There is, too, the 'Kiss of the Upper Lip' in which the man kisses the woman's upper lip and she in turn kisses his lower lip. A 'Clasping Kiss' is when one partner takes both lips of the other between her or his lips. Kisses in which tongues entwine and mingle deeply, touching the inside of the mouth and the palate, are called 'Fighting of the Tongue'.

The next section of the Kama Sutra deals with a slightly more sophisticated element of love-making - scratching with the fingernails, biting with the teeth and striking with the palm of the hands or the fists.

All the ancient books of love and sex instruction from the East include sections on scratching and biting and, indeed, the fingernails were an important cosmetic detail for sexually active people.

The most delicate technique, and one preferred when the female partner is just a young girl, is called 'Sounding', which simply

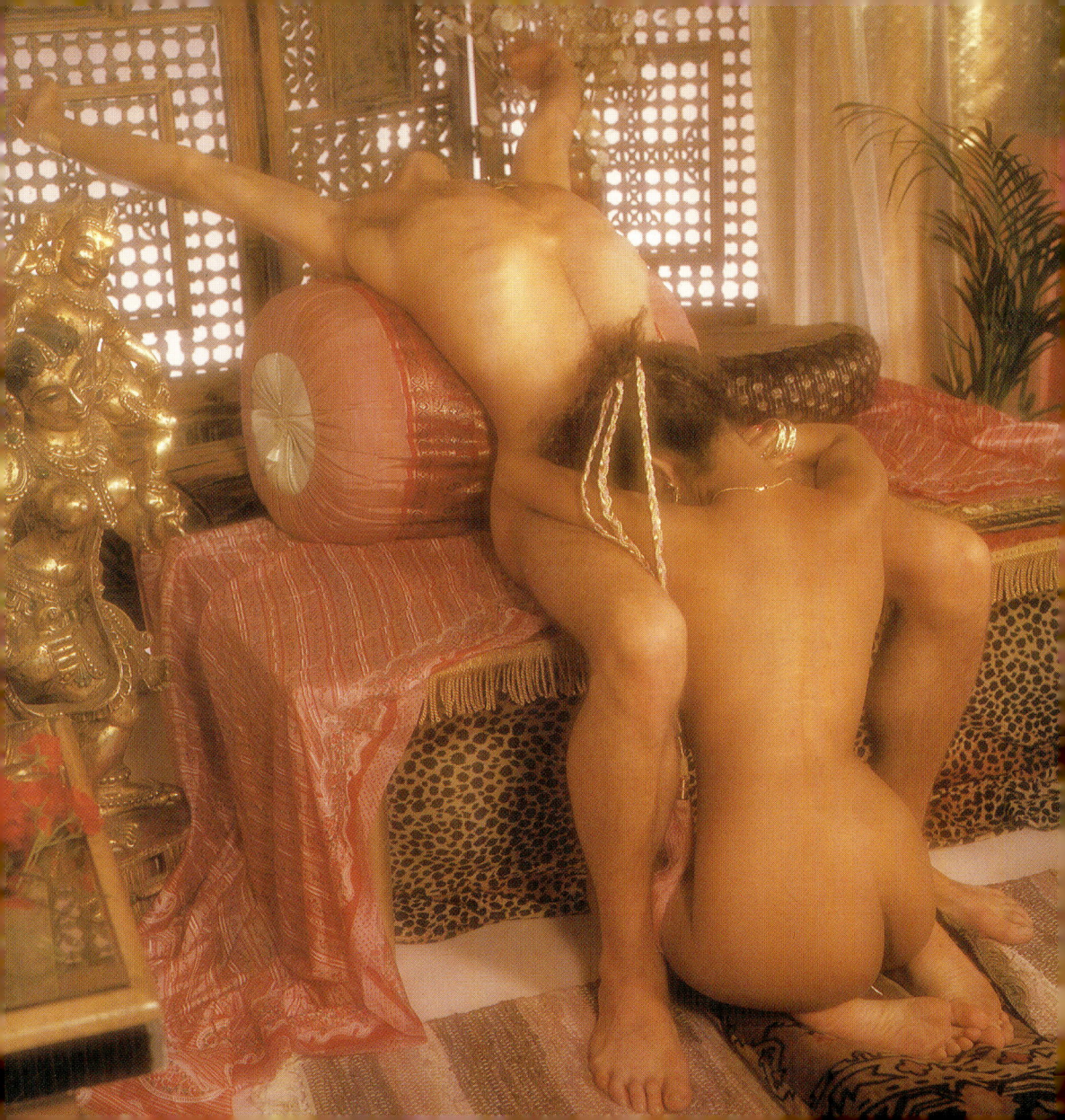

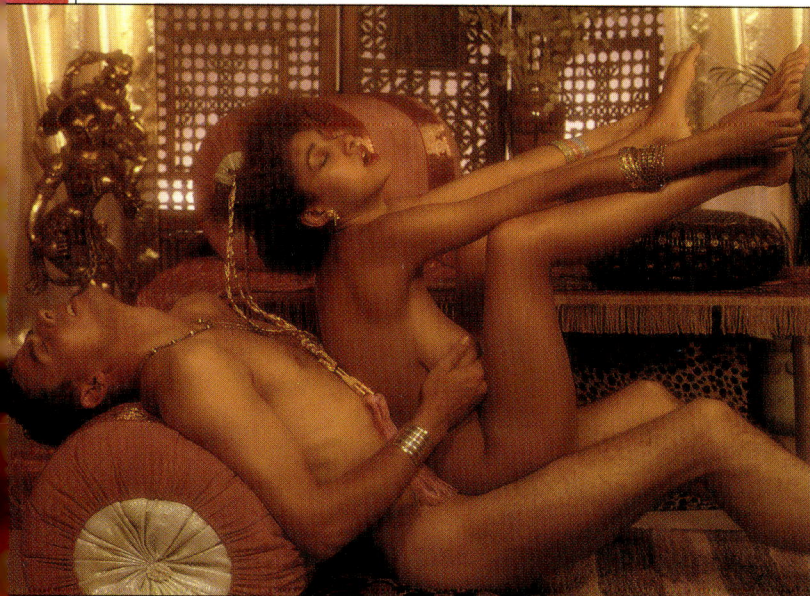

means pressing with the nails very softly and without leaving any mark. A single curved mark left by a deeper pressure is called a 'Half-moon', and two half moons opposite each other are a 'Circle'. There are several other marks specified, each with its own particular name. A curved mark made with all five nails, and left on the breast, is called the 'Peacock's Foot' and a note adds that a great deal of skill is required to be able to do it properly and that those who do it are, therefore, seeking notice and praise.

Part of the function of scratching and biting seems to

To allow her partner to rest, the *Kama Sutra* advises the woman to take over 'the work of the man' from time to time, that is, position herself on top.

have been to draw public notice to the fact that a love affair was going on. A young woman showing love bites or nail marks on her breast or throat was an object of admiration. However, such visible marks were not deemed suitable for married women - though certain private marks could be made. Love marks acted as reminders for the participants, too. It was considered appropriate for a man to mark his wife or lover in this way when he was about to go on a journey, so that she would remember him.

The same instructions apply to love bites. Eight kinds of bite are listed, and for a lover to achieve his desired effect some skill would be needed to make very precise patterns.

Among the bites, interestingly, is the 'Biting of a Boar', which consists of several broad rows of marks near to one another with red intervals. This is made on the breasts and shoulders and is particularly associated with highly passionate people. The 'Hidden Bite', which just leaves the skin red, is made specially on the lower lip and the 'String of Points', when small sections of skin are bitten with all the teeth, can be done on the throat, the armpit and the joints of the thighs.

Finally, the author suggests that when a man bites a woman then she should return the compliment twice as strongly, offering two bruises to his one and so forth. She is also invited to start a love quarrel and then conclude it by grabbing him by the hair, shutting her eyes and biting him in various places.

Sexual intercourse can be compared to a quarrel, remarks Vatsyayana at one point, because of the contrarieties of love and its tendency to dispute. Also, high passion can inspire lovers to strike each other, literally. There are four kinds of blow - that with the back of the hand, that with the fingers a little contracted, that with the fist and that with the

Many positions for the 'woman on top' are described. The 'Spin' and the 'Swing' are famous, but less athletic variants are also popular.

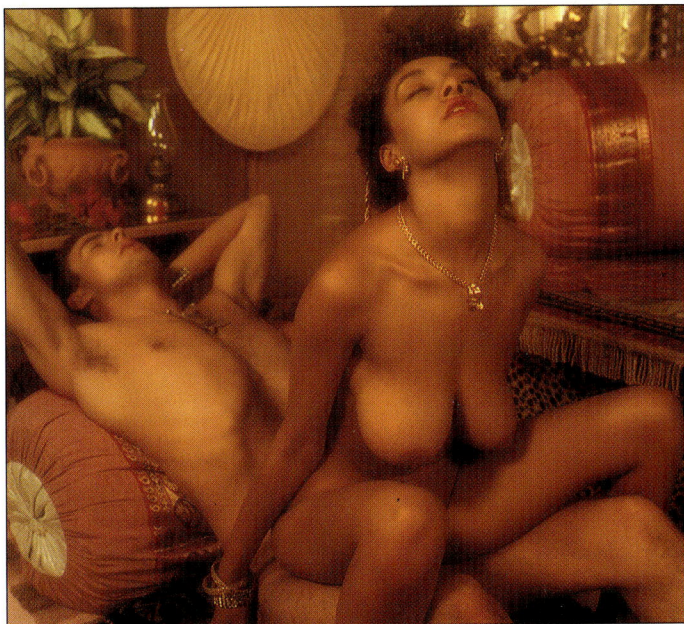

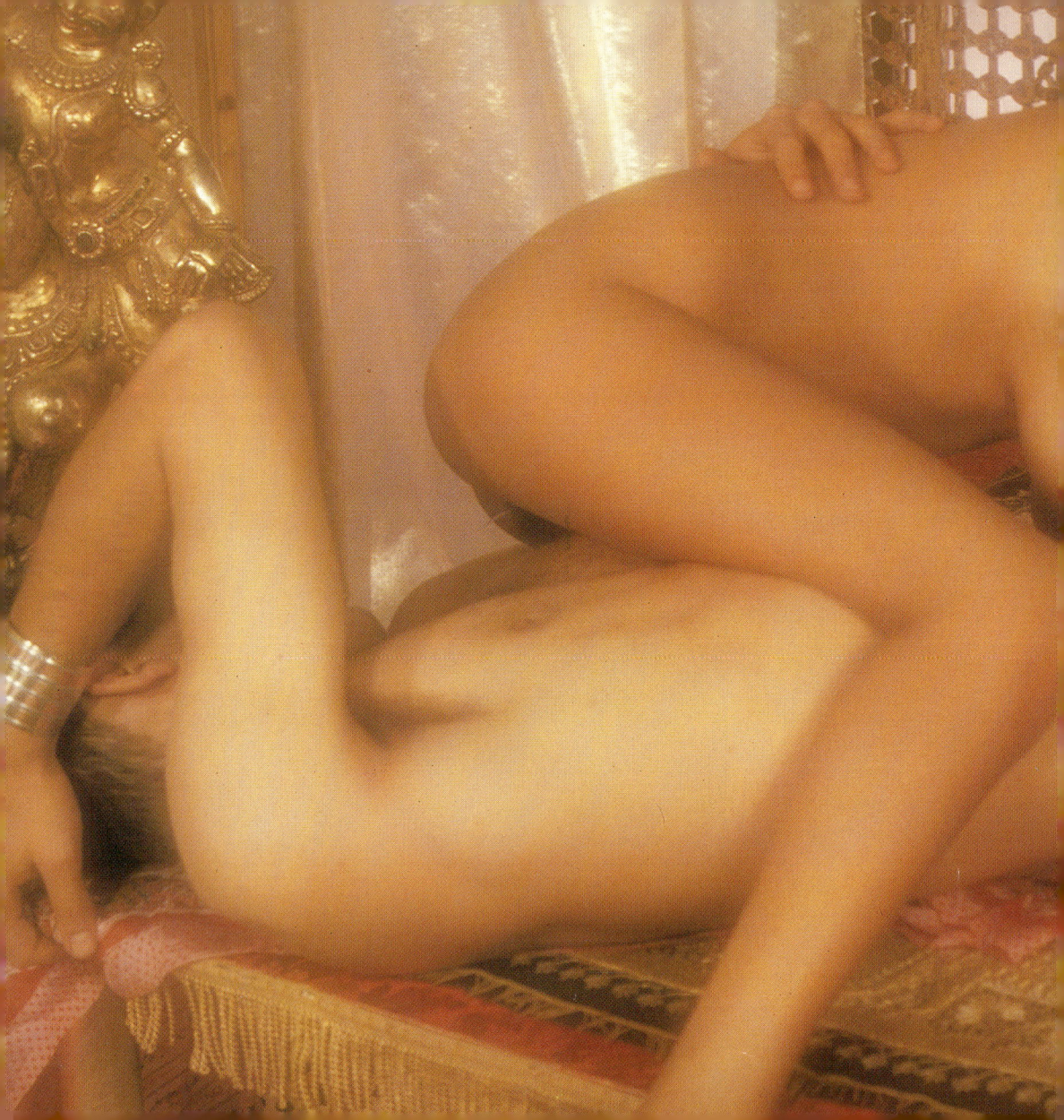

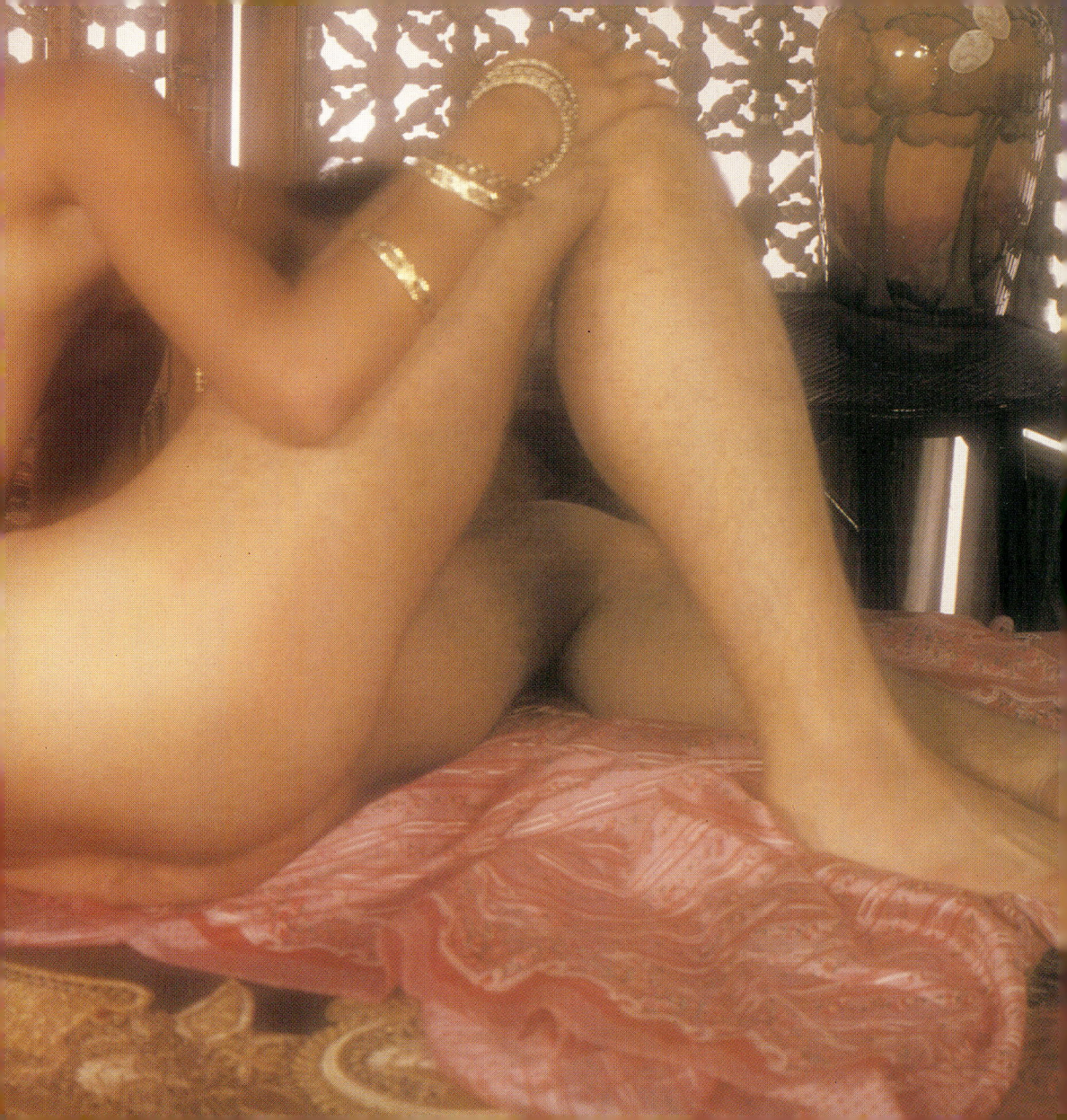

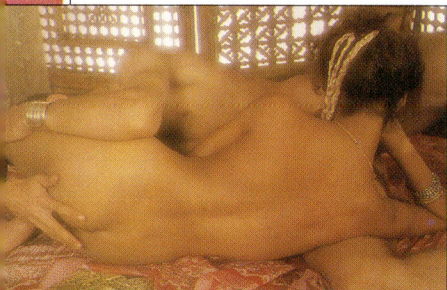

open palm of the hand. The special parts of the body for striking are the shoulders, the head, the space betweeen the breasts, the back, the middle part of the body and the sides. There are also particular sounds associated with each kind of blow, a litany of noises expressing pain, praise, a request to stop, or a request for more: and it is suggested that noises like those made by birds (parrot, sparrow, flamingo, etc.) could be used. And while the woman is being made love to, the space between her breasts should be struck with the back of the hand, slowly at first but faster and faster as the excitement of intercourse increases.

The Positions of Love

As we have seen, the Kama Sutra describes the caressing and stimulating actions and gestures which a loving couple might use in ritualistic detail. Distinction is made between techniques designed to turn a man or woman on, and those which can be used when passion is running high for a variety or just for fun.

The section devoted to positions recommended for sexual union is, perhaps, the most celebrated passage in the Kama Sutra: to Western eyes many of them seem uncomfortable, too athletic to achieve, and difficult, if not impossible. Yet at the same

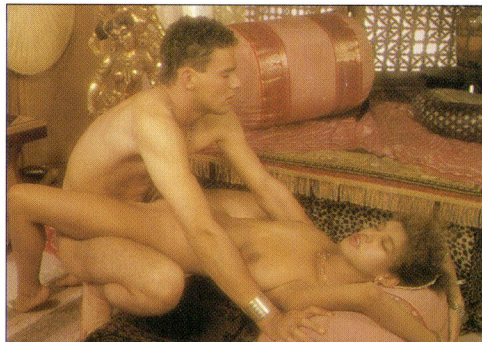

Once more, the woman does 'the work of the man', this time with the extra support of cushions. This is a variation on the 'Pair of Tongs' position, shown later.

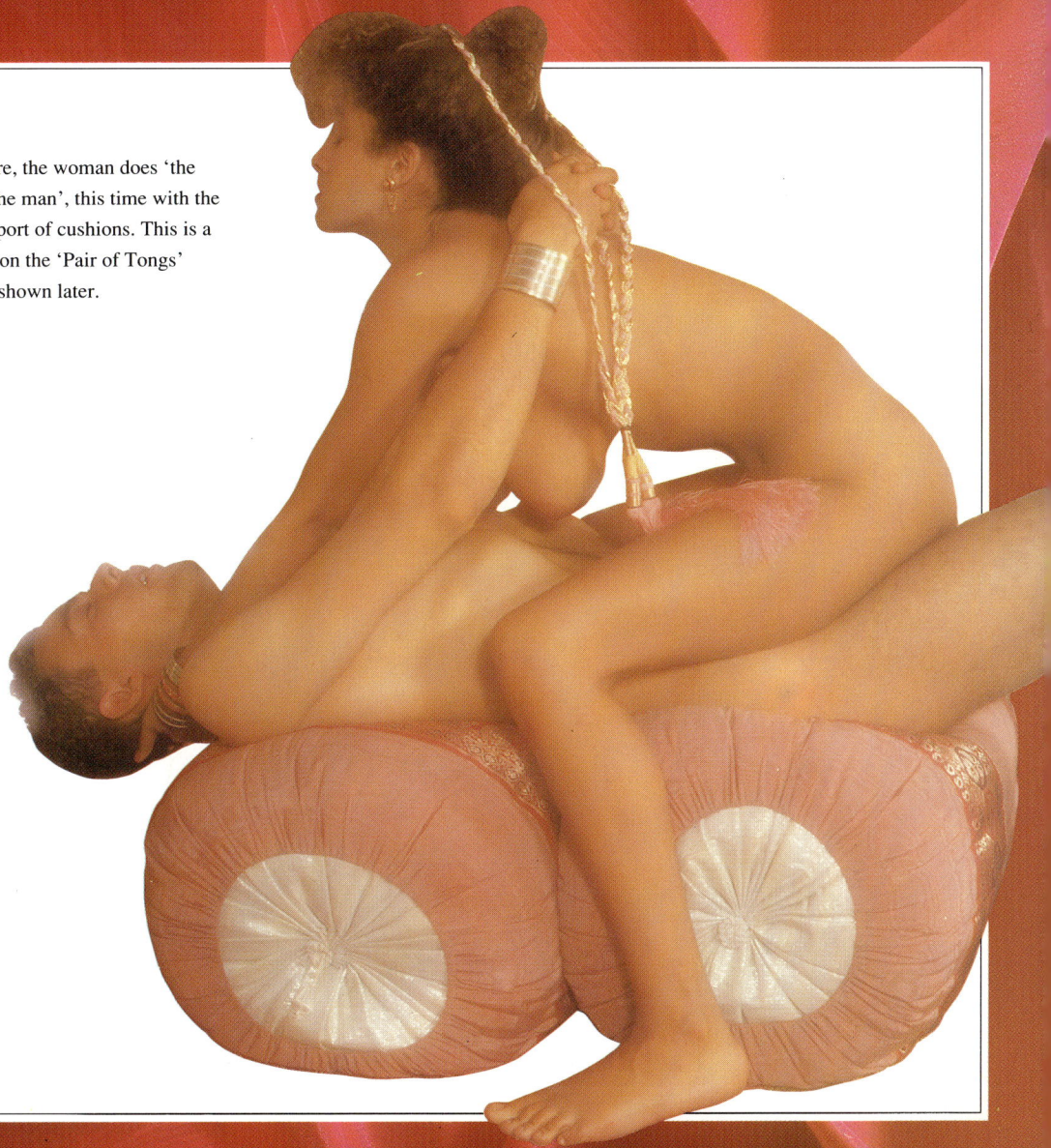

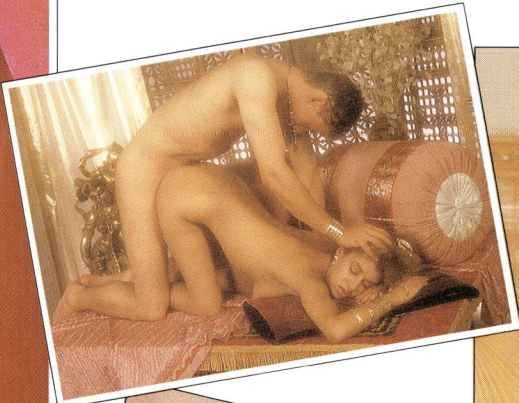

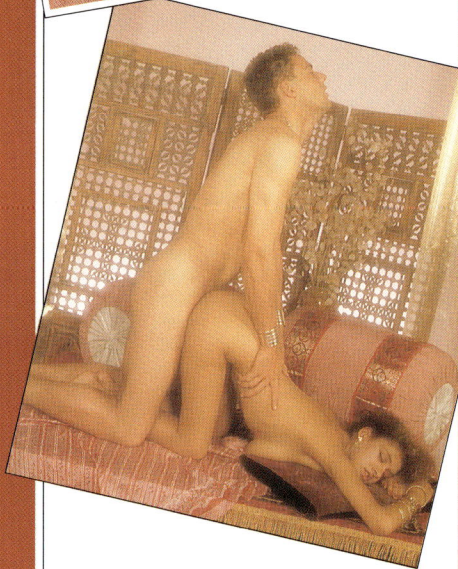

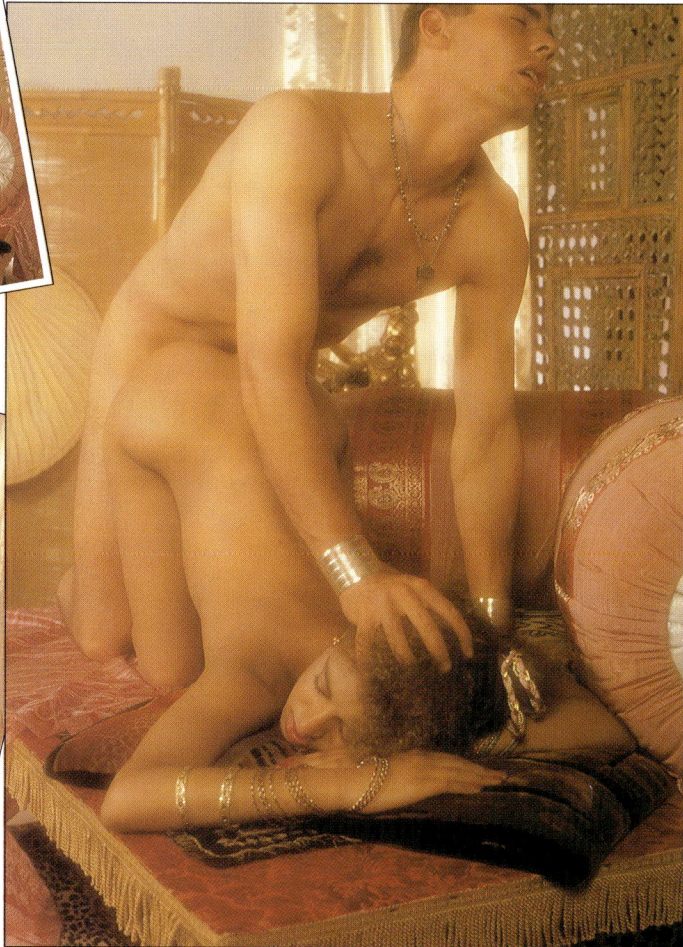

time they remain deeply exciting and suggest the possibilities of fluid, flexible, ecstatic and - above all - equal kinds of union.

Discussing 'various kinds of congress', Vatsyayana returns immediately to the point with which he started his discourse on the practicalities of sex: genital size. And the first three positions he offers concern the deer-woman (who has the smallest yoni). She may adopt the 'Widely Open Position', the 'Yawning Position' or the 'Position of the Wife of Indra'. All these positions are designed to help her widen her yoni to accommodate a larger than appropriate lingam.

WIDELY OPEN POSITION: The woman lies back, lowers her head and raises her middle part towards the man, who may kneel or squat between her legs.

THE YAWNING POSITION: Here she lies back, raises her thighs and keeps them wide apart throughout love-making.

POSITION OF THE WIFE OF INDRA, OR THE 'INDRANI' POSITION: The woman lies back and draws her thighs up so that her knees are close against her flanks. This position, the book notes, is quite different and must be learned through practise. Certainly, to draw the thighs back and keep them pressed against the body in this way does demand a certain flexibility, though in practise pressure from the man's own body would help the woman to maintain the position.

The next three positions described are particularly suitable for those occasions when the woman's yoni is too deep to match the size of the man's lingam.

THE CLASPING POSITION: The woman lies flat on her back, her arms stretched out beyond her head. The man lies directly on

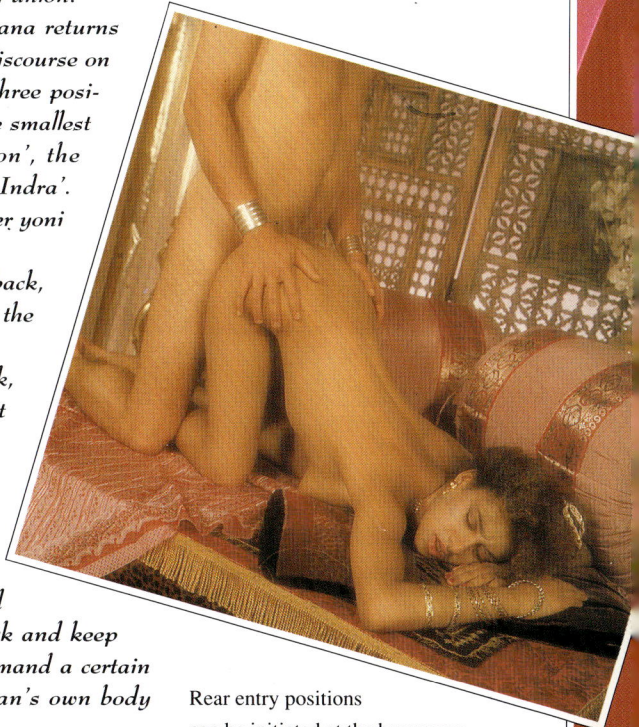

Rear entry positions can be initiated at the beginning of intercourse or, if the couple are supple and active enough, may be the climax of the 'Turning Position'.

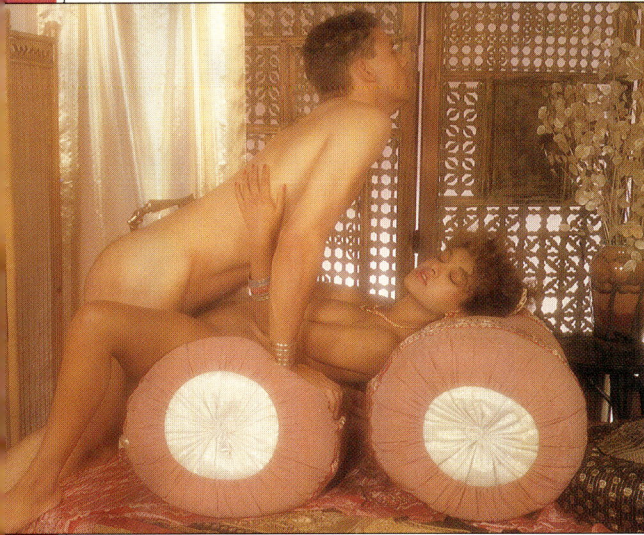

The *Kama Sutra* does not view making love as lying down on the job. Many positions are listed which can be enjoyed standing up, leaning against walls, or supported by various props. Squatting, sitting, crouching, kneeling and leaning were all acceptable postures by either partner.

top of her, with all parts of his body from legs to hands touching hers as far as possible. If the man is taller than the woman, then a cushion placed at her feet will support his feet at the appropriate height. This position can also be done with the couple lying on their sides, facing each other.

THE PRESSING POSITION: This is an extension of the previous position. Once lovemaking has begun and the lingam has been inserted into the yoni, then the woman should bring her thighs together as tightly as possible, thus holding the lingam firmly in place.

THE MARE'S POSITION: The woman brings her legs tightly together and forcibly holds the lingam in her yoni. The manual remarks that this is difficult and learned through practice, but doesn't make it clear exactly how the lingam is 'forcibly' held - by hand or the vagina.

THE RISING POSITION: The female lies back and raises her thighs straight up. She can be sitting on her partner's thighs and he can assist by holding her thighs.

YAWNING POSITION II: Here she raises her legs and places them on her lover's shoulders.

PRESSED POSITION: Here she bends her knees, raises her legs and presses her feet against the chest of her lover. By clasping her round the thighs he can pull her very close towards him.

HALF-PRESSED POSITION: One foot is pressed against the man's chest as in the previous position, but the other leg is allowed to stretch out around him.

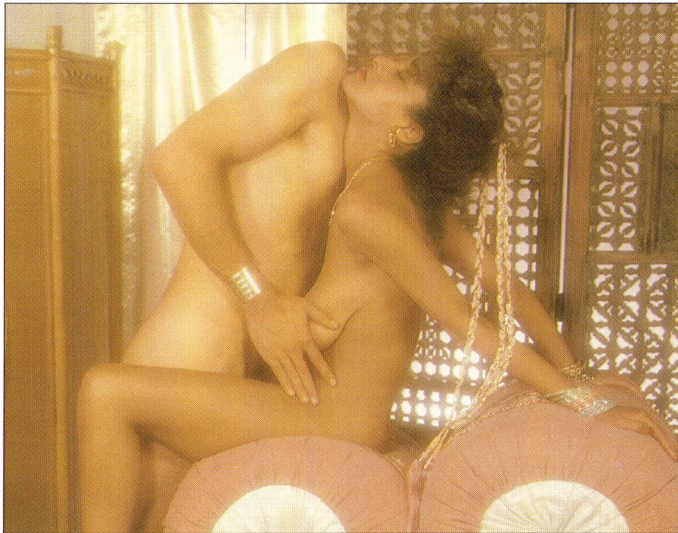

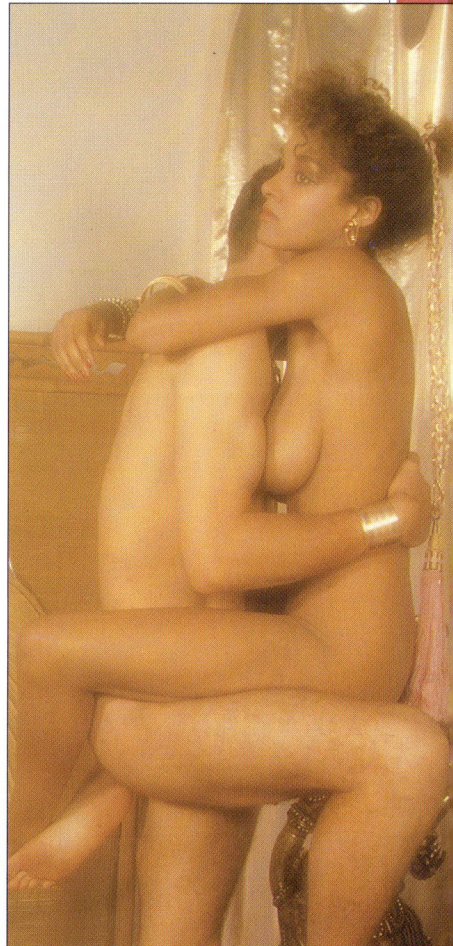

SPLITTING BAMBOO: So far, the positions listed have been fairly straightforward and designed to make the best accommodation between lingams and yonis of various sizes. Now we move into a more elaborate area. For this position, the woman lies back, places one leg on her lover's shoulder and stretches the other leg right out. Then she reverses the procedure and changes the position of her legs alternately while congress is proceeding. The alternate stretching and bending of the legs would create exciting ripples and changes in the position and muscular tension of the yoni, and a change of position of the legs would need to coincide with each thrust of the lingam. Thus, each time the man thrusts inwards the woman would change the angles of her legs, and again

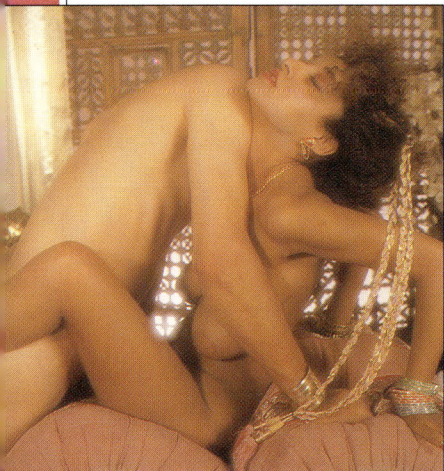

as he withdraws. Obviously, this needs concentration and practice.

FIXING A NAIL: The woman lies back and places one of her legs so that the foot rests on the nape of her neck. The other leg is stretched out. Obviously, to achieve this a woman needs to be very flexible indeed and the Kama Sutra does state that this is 'learned by practice only'.

THE CRAB: When both the legs of the woman are contracted and the feet are fixed firmly on the regions of her stomach.

THE PACKED POSITION: This is another position which is intended to ensure a tight fit of lingam into yoni. The woman lies back, raises her thighs and then crosses her legs at the ankles.

THE LOTUS-LIKE POSITION: This incorporates the lotus posture of the yogi. The woman lies and crosses her legs in the lotus position - but with the legs raised up to her breasts.

THE TURNING POSITION: The act of intercourse may start in any position provided the man can slowly turn around and, moving the woman as he does so, eventually enjoy her from behind without withdrawing his lingam from her yoni. Clearly this requires practice, but with the willing cooperation of the woman it is not quite so arduous as it may sound.

All the positions described so far require the couple to be lying down or reclining in some way.

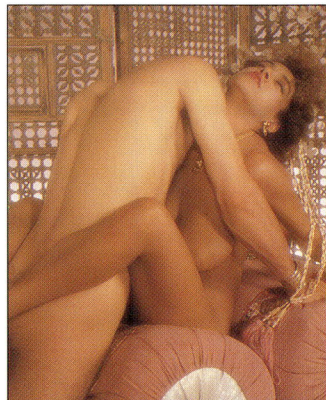

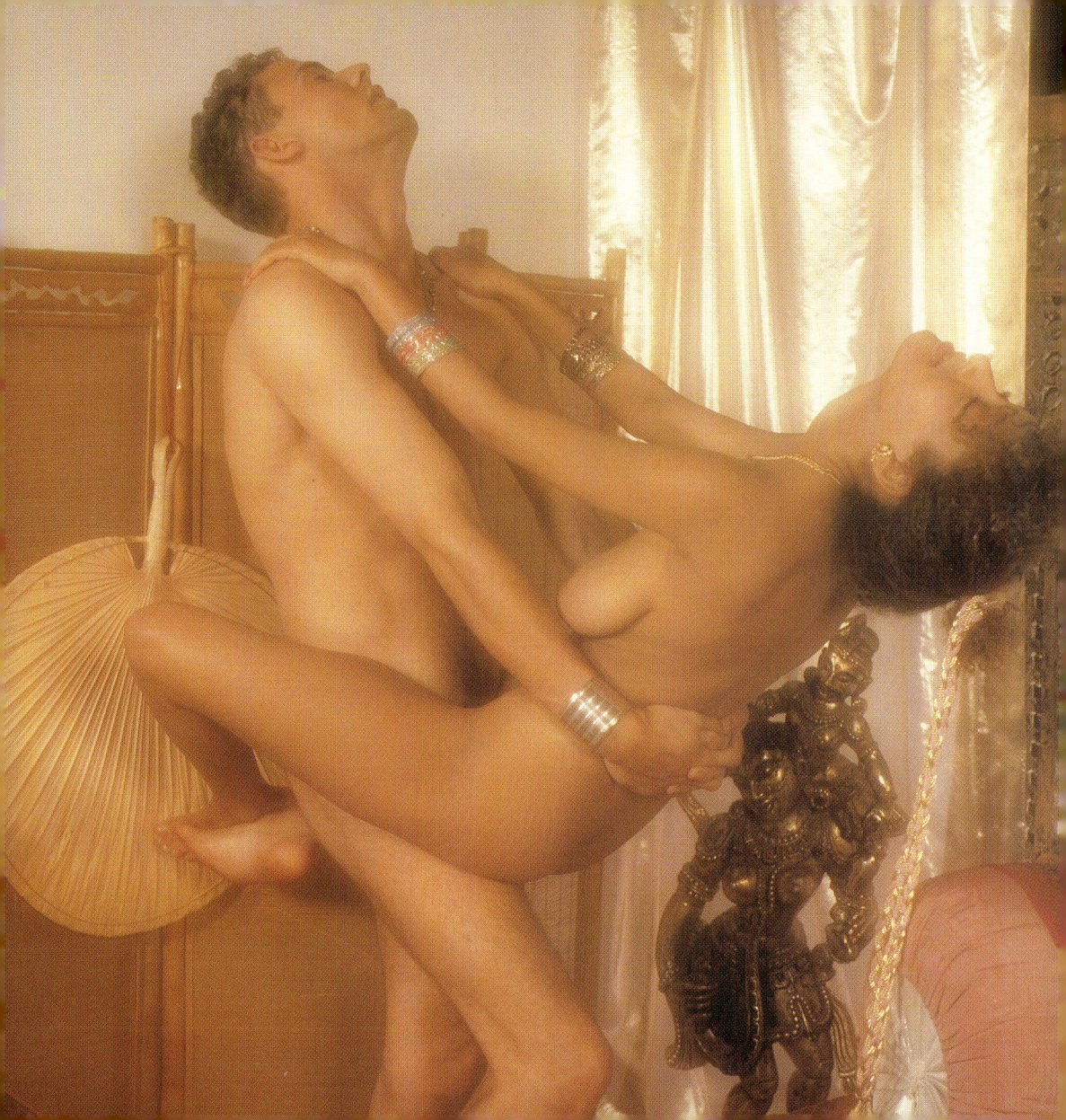

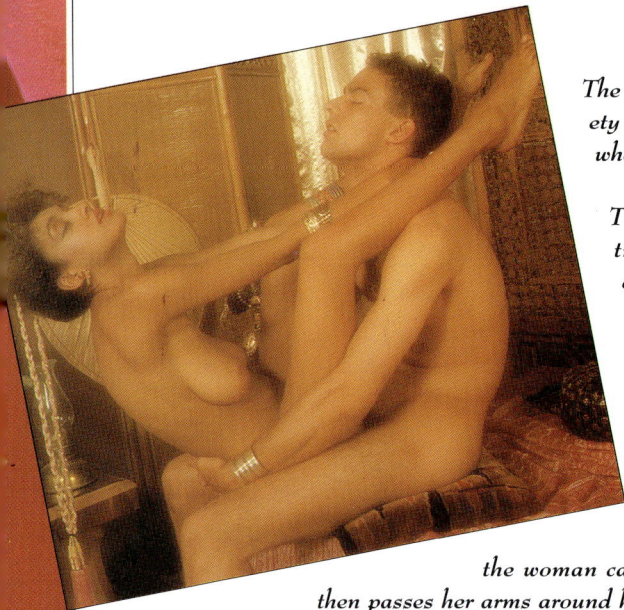

The Kama Sutra *now looks at the variety of positions available to the couple when they are standing up.*

THE SUPPORTED POSITION: This is the basic standing-up position. The couple can support each other with their own bodies or they can lean against a wall. Almost any comfortable variation of previously described sexual positions may be used.

SUSPENDED POSITION: The man supports himself against a wall or pillar and clasps his hands together so that the woman can sit on them as on a swing. She then passes her arms around his neck and raises her thighs to his waist-level, resting her feet against the wall or pillar. When the couple are sure of their balance, she can move herself up and down on his lingam by pushing with her feet.

ANIMAL POSITIONS: A number of postures are named after the congress of particular animals - cows, goats, deer, horses, tigers and elephants, etc.

The various 'animal' postures are all variations of the rear-entry positions - not anal intercourse but, rather, approaching the yoni from behind. The woman might simply bend over, she might get down on all fours, she may lie on her face. These positions all ensure the maximum exposure of the yoni and ease of its access to the lingam. They need full co-operation from the woman.

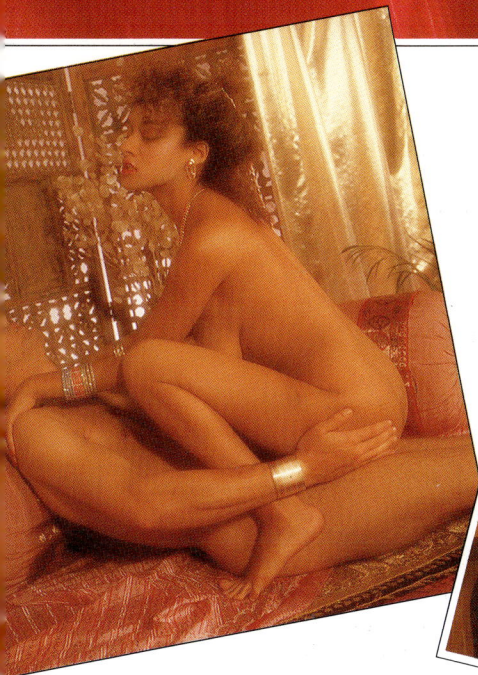

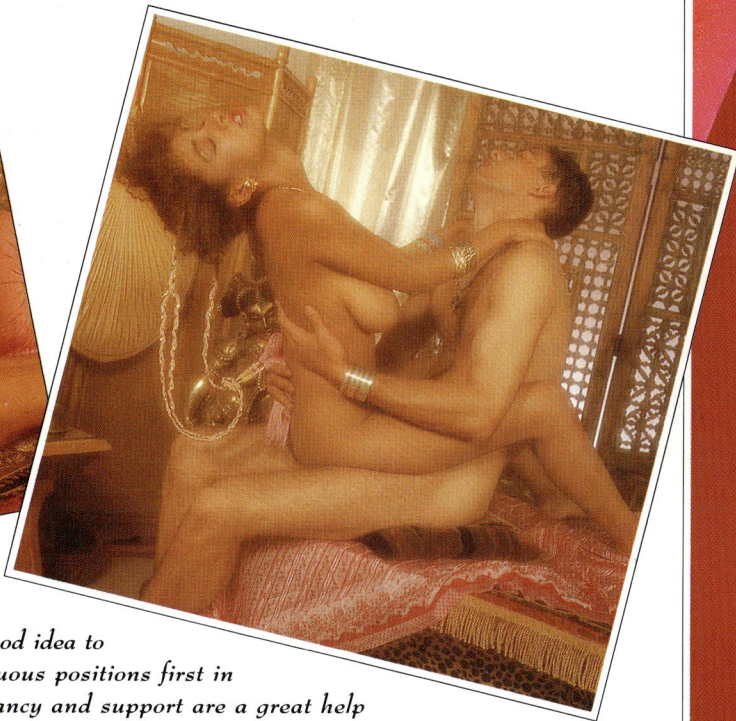

The Kama Sutra
suggests that it is a good idea to
practise the more arduous positions first in
water, since the buoyancy and support are a great help
when trying new body postures.

But despite the demands made on the female partner, it
remains clear that the man was required to use rather more sheer
physical energy in love-making. Most of the time he is not merely
doing the thrusting but also helping to support his partner by holding her waist, thighs or back in the chosen position. And the Kama
Sutra realises that a man may occasionally a get a little tired,
especially if intercourse has been going on for some time and he
hasn't yet reached a climax.

The 'work of a man' as it is called, remains as effective a model for efficient lovemaking today as it was when it was compiled.

If the woman is a virgin, the man is advised first to get his hands on her breasts, which she will probably try to keep covered. He must do this gently but persuasively. Such a young girl will also probably keep her thighs pressed closely together and, again, it is the business of the man to place his hands between her thighs and slowly work them apart.

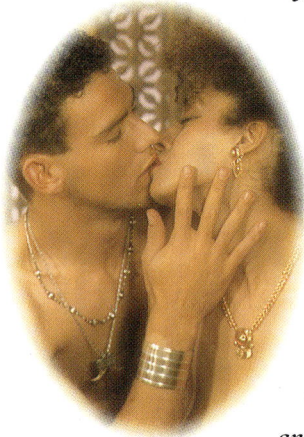

If his partner is a seasoned woman, says the text briskly, then they can do whatever it is that pleases them most. But whoever the woman is, the man is urged to take his cue from her, to touch those parts of her body 'on which she turns her eyes' and to realise from her gestures and attitudes what particular parts of her body she would most like caressed.

There follow nine separate ways in which the male should move his lingam in intercourse. 'Moving Forward' is when the organs are brought together directly and he slides straight in. 'Churning' is when he holds his lingam in his hand and turns it in the yoni. 'Piercing' is when the yoni is lowered and the upper part is struck with the lingam. 'Rubbing' is the same but done to the lower part of the yoni. 'Pressing' is when the lingam is inserted deeply into the yoni and pressed firmly inside. When the lingam is removed a little way out of the yoni and then thrust back firmly to strike it, it is called 'Giving a Blow'. When only one part of the yoni is rubbed by the lingam it is called the 'Blow of a Boar', and the 'Blow of a Bull' involves rubbing both sides of the yoni in much the same way.

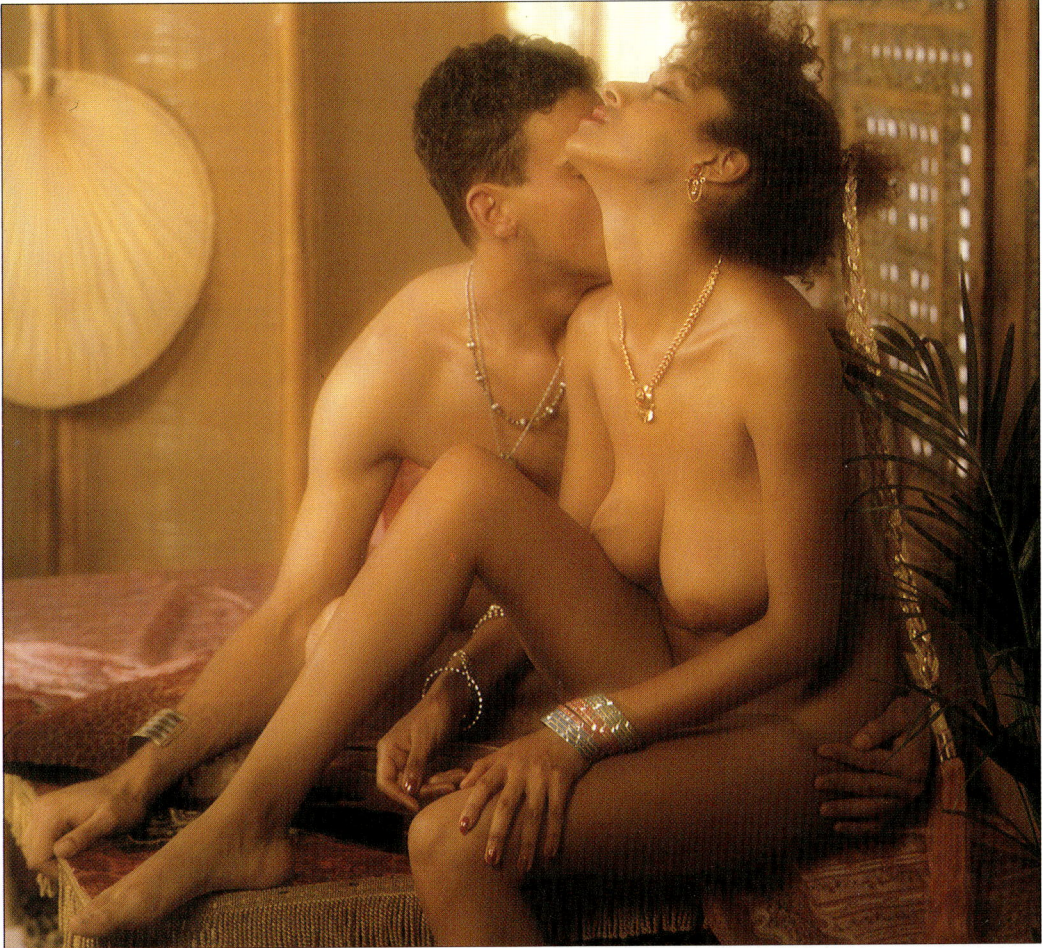

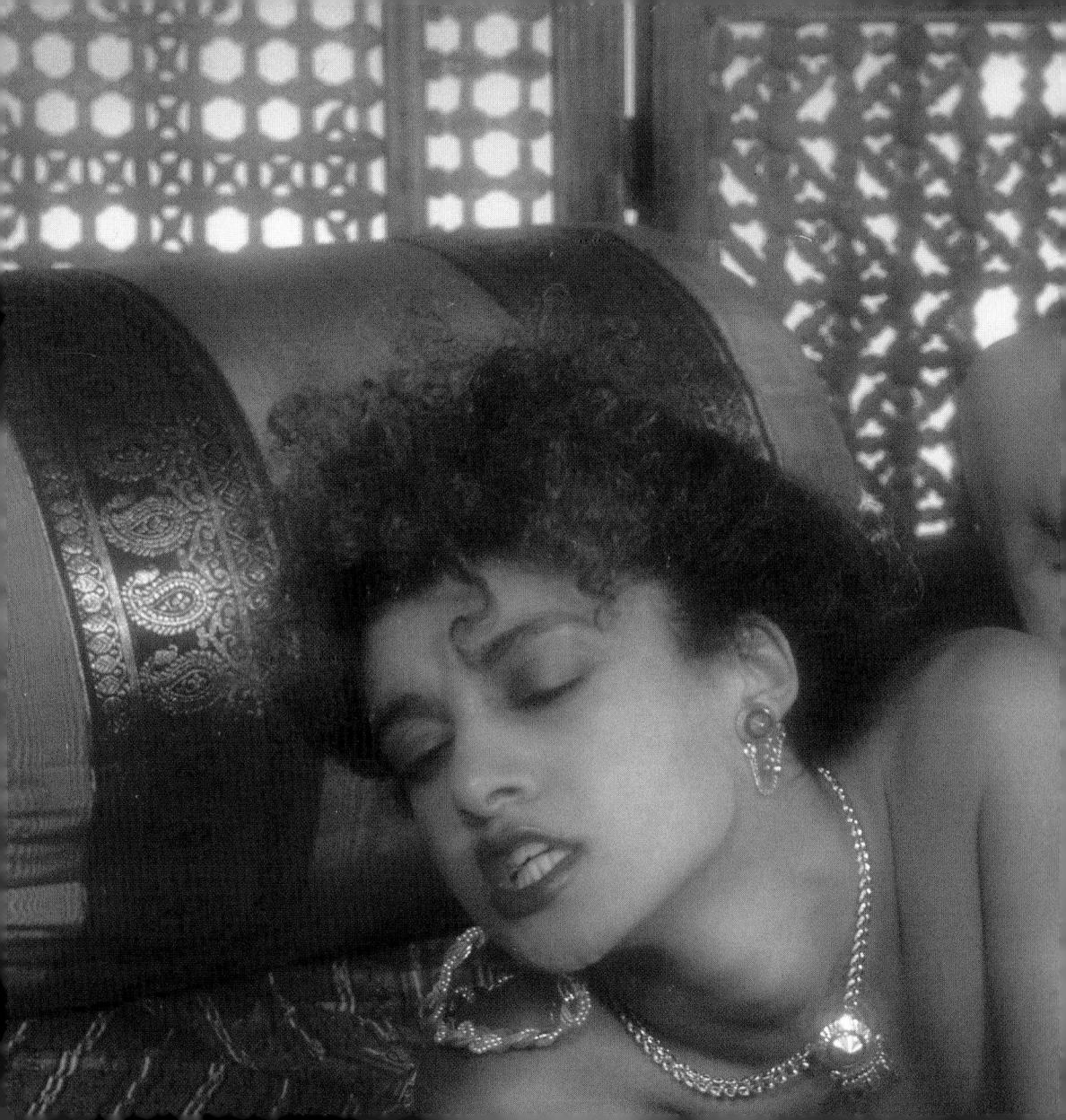

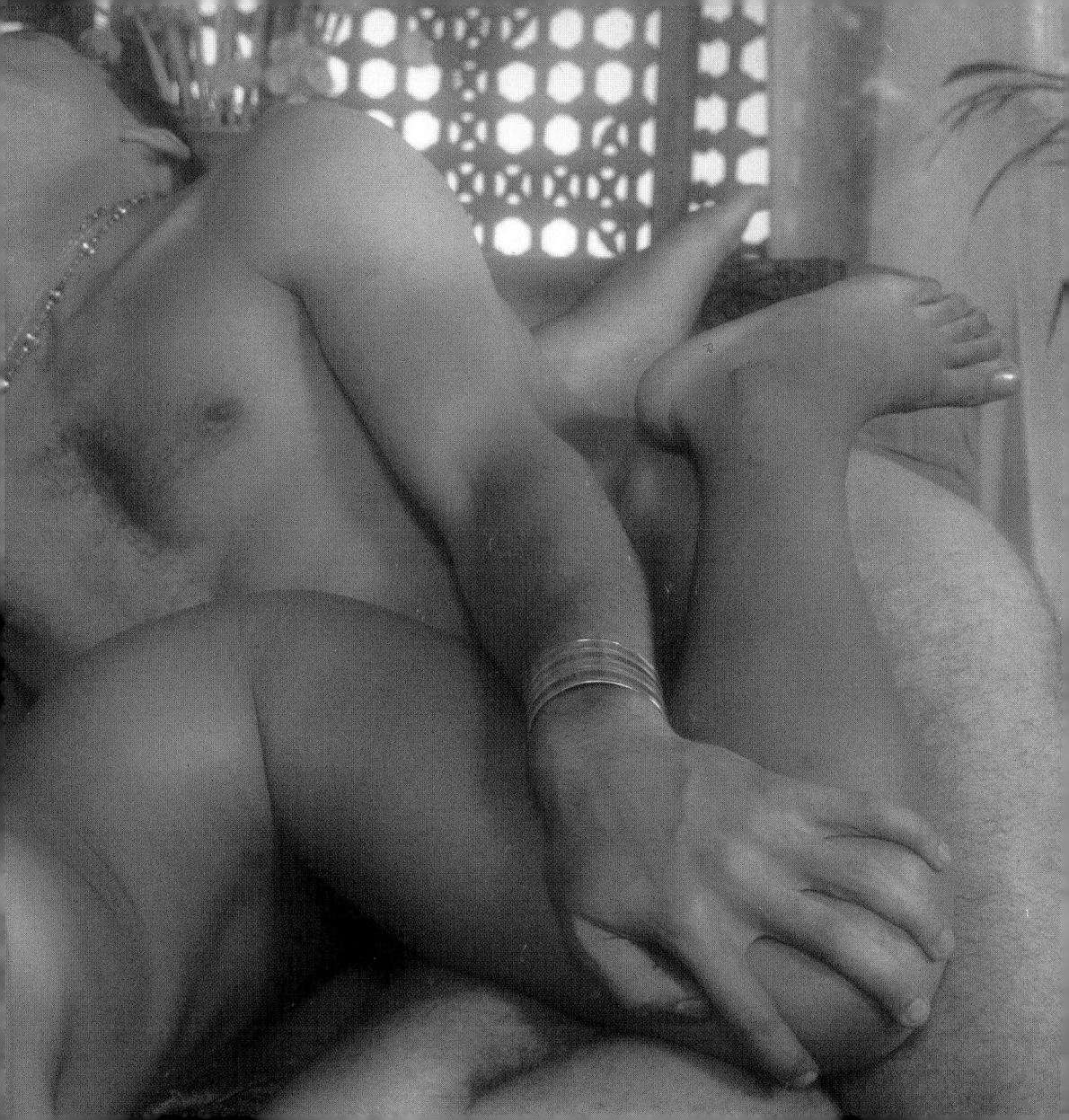

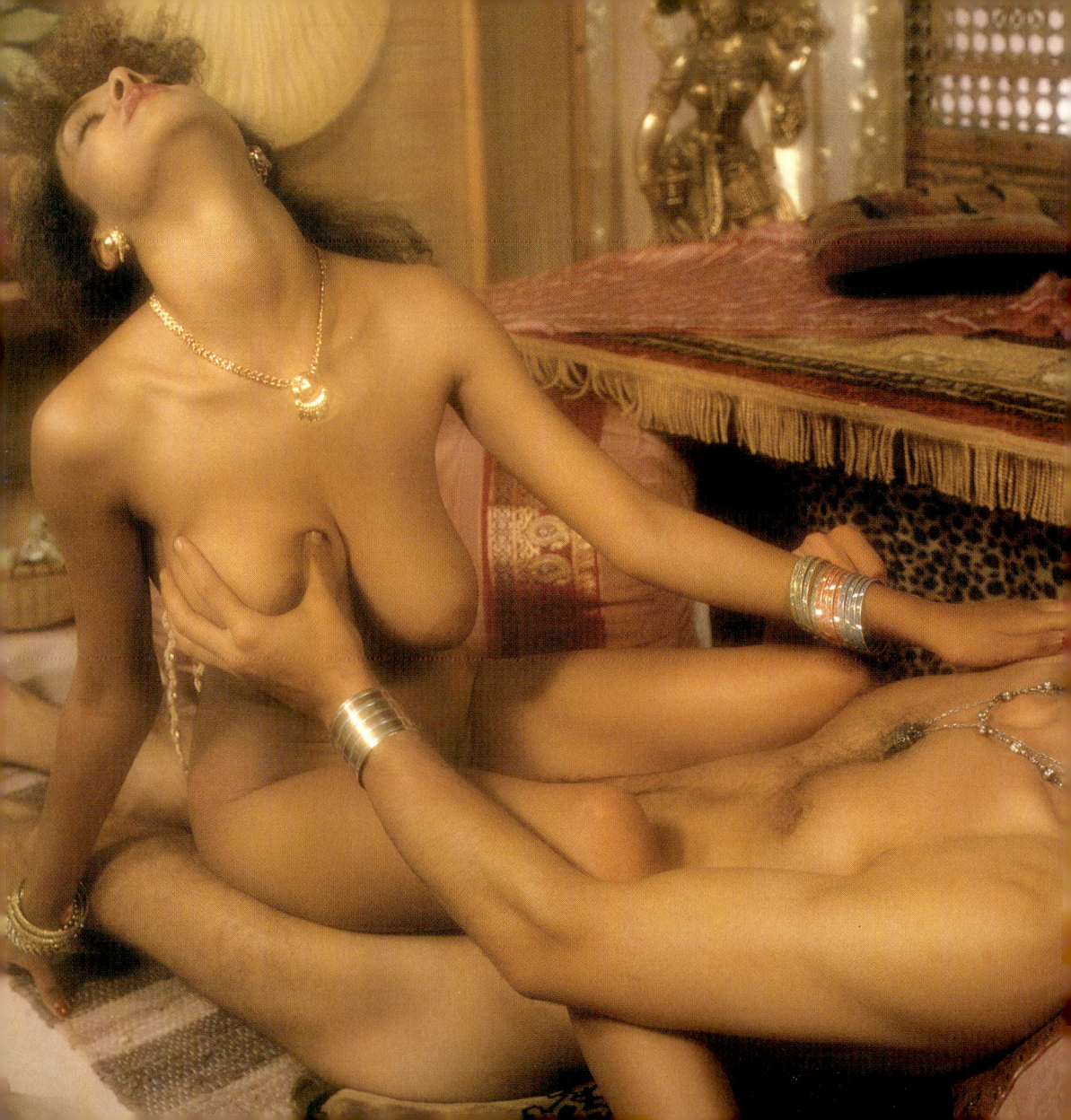

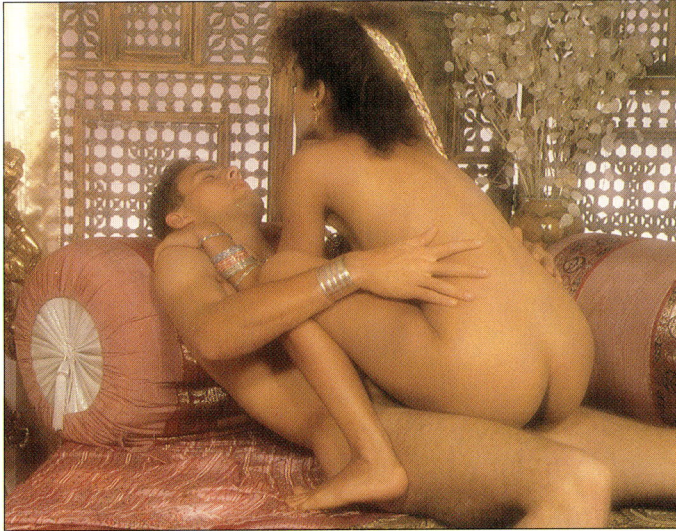

The 'Sporting of a Sparrow' happens when the lingam is right inside the yoni and is moved up and down quickly but without being removed at all. This is recommended for the last phases of intercourse and promotes the man's orgasm fairly quickly.

If a woman perceives that her lover is getting a little tired, it is suggested that she should take over the 'work of a man' for a while. She must lay him on his back and proceed to act his part, using as many of the gestures and techniques outlined above as are suitable for her. Positions available to her are:

THE PAIR OF TONGS: She squats or sits on top of him, drawing him into her, and holds his lingam inside by the pressure of her thighs for a long time.

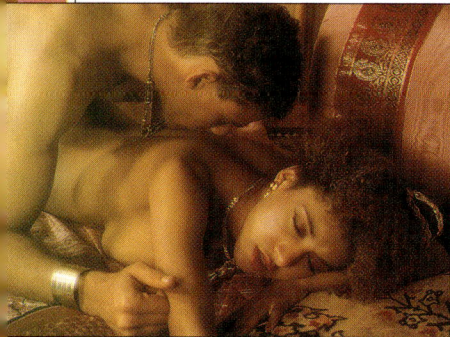

THE SPINNING TOP: *This is possibly the most famous of all the Kama Sutra positions and involves the woman turning herself round on top of the man while keeping his lingam firmly inside her. This probably needs full participation from the male and is best attempted with him lying or half-reclining on the floor. But the man can raise the central part of his body up in a kind of arch, resting on his hands and feet. The woman is then poised above him to begin her spins. Good balance is essential.*

THE SWING: *This is a slightly more accessible version of the Spinning Top. Again the male raises his body in an arc and the woman impales herself on his erect lingam - but turned around so that her back is facing him. She then rocks back and forward, maintaining her balance and control by keeping her feet in contact with the ground.*

The chapter on oral sex is probably the most ambiguous section of the Kama Sutra. It is firmly related to the male; to the sucking of the lingam. It was not seen as a part of regular, straightforward lovemaking but rather as a specialist function of the art of massage.

The sequence for the oral caress of the lingam begins with the shaft being held in the hand and the tip gently brushed between the lips. The sides may then be pressed with the lips and the teeth used, but delicately. The lingam is again inserted into the mouth and kissed as if it were the lower

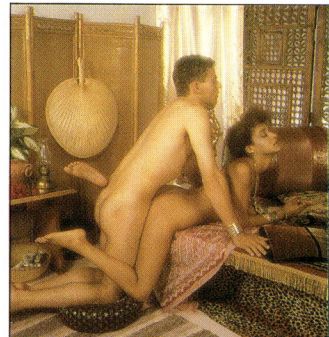

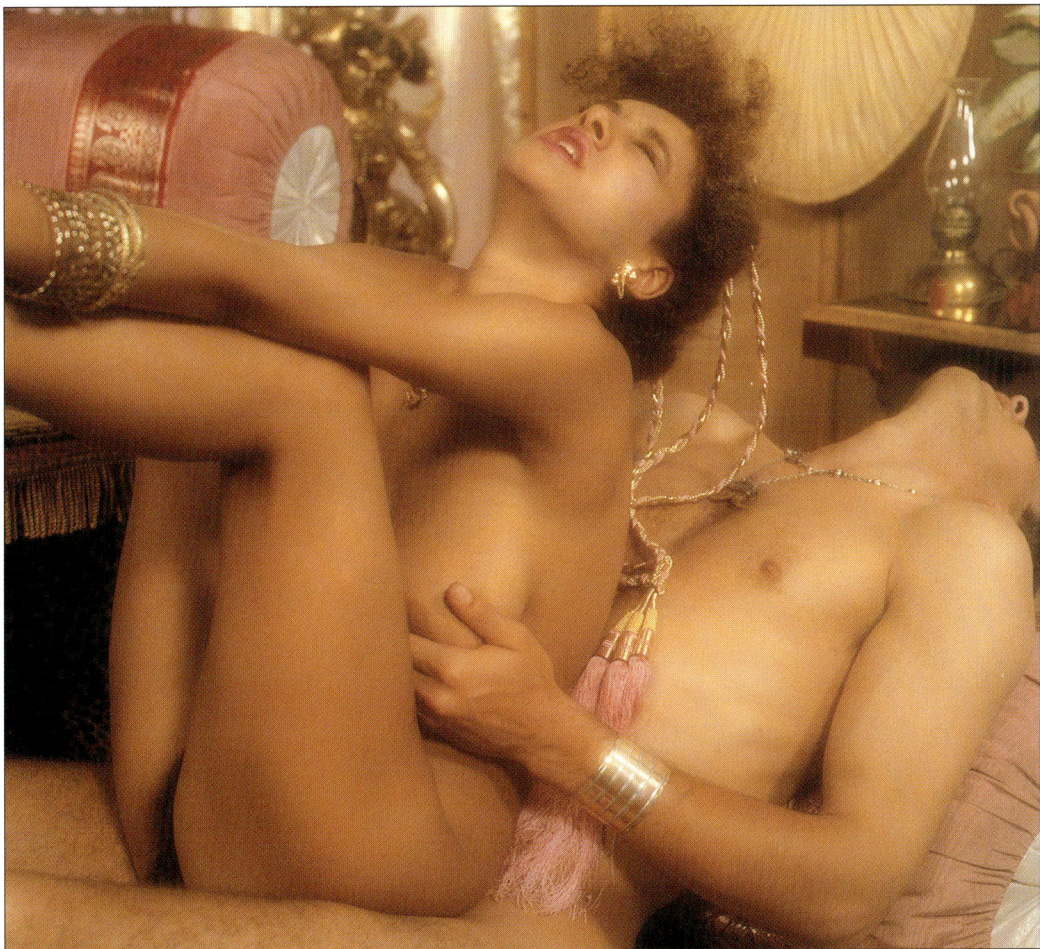

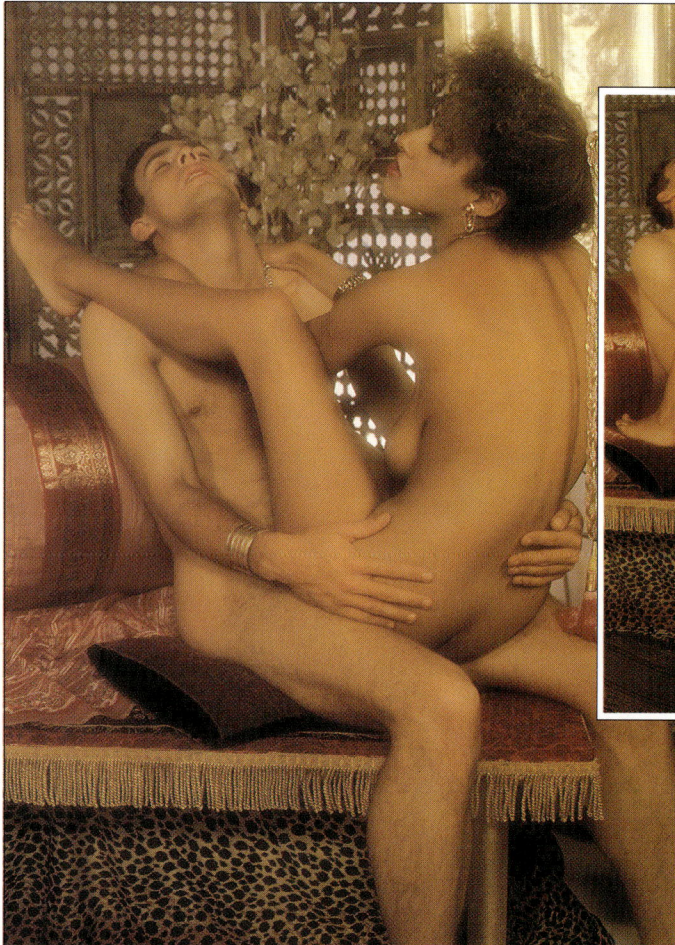

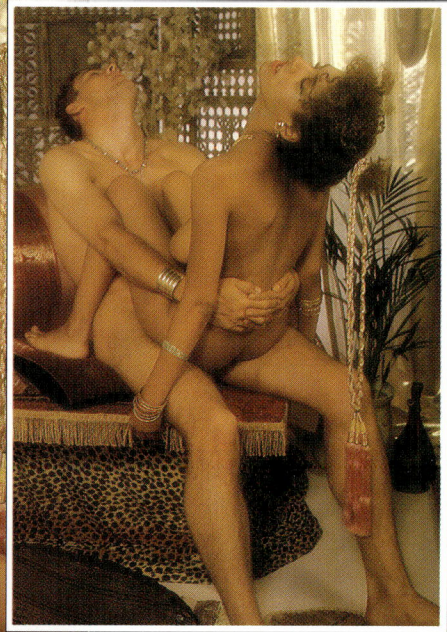

Nowhere in the *Kama Sutra* is there any sense of the woman lying back, closing her eyes and waiting for something to be done to her. Women were seen as fully cooperating partners in lovemaking.

lips of a lover; it is then licked all over (including the tip) by the tongue, then put halfway into the mouth and forcefully kissed and sucked. Finally, it is drawn completely into the mouth pressed in to the end as far as it will go and sucked as if being swallowed. This last action is what we call 'Deep Throat'.

Instructions for kissing the yoni are almost brutally brief. 'The way of doing this should be known from kissing the mouth'. One particular position is mentioned - the 'Congress of the Crow', which is what we would call 69, with the couple inverted so each may caress the other's genitals with their mouth. This can be performed lying or standing.

This ends the section of the Kama Sutra which is devoted exclusively to sexual activity and techniques. It is all-embracing and covers almost every aspect of the subject, making it as relevant today as it was when first written.

Little Extras

The Kama Sutra includes passages on what we would call sex aids, and contains lists of recipes for aphrodisiacs and other love potions - that is, concoctions designed to arouse sexual passion in oneself and concoctions designed to make other people find one desirable.

Whether these potions literally worked is obviously doubtful, but the correct creation of aphrodisiacs and love potions was a specialised branch of Indian medicine and had religious approval. It is possible that the ointments and unguents which were rubbed

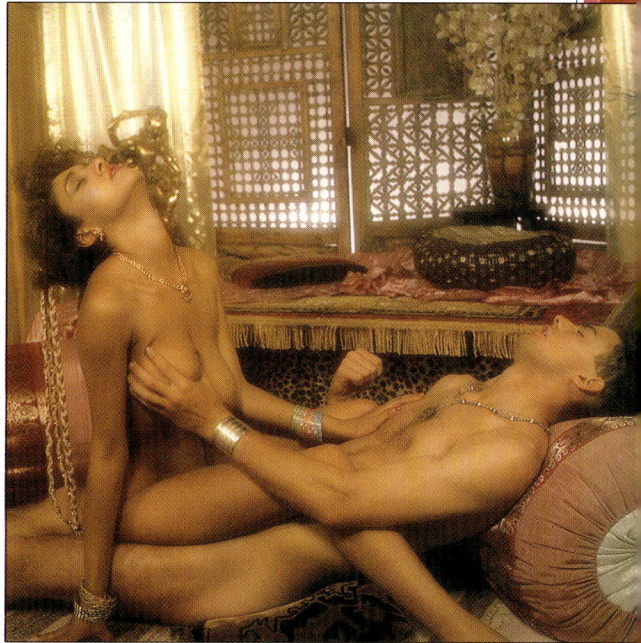

A simple ritual is described for use when the woman became tired in her turn. She leans forward and places her forehead against her lover's and, without releasing his lingam, ceases her movements.

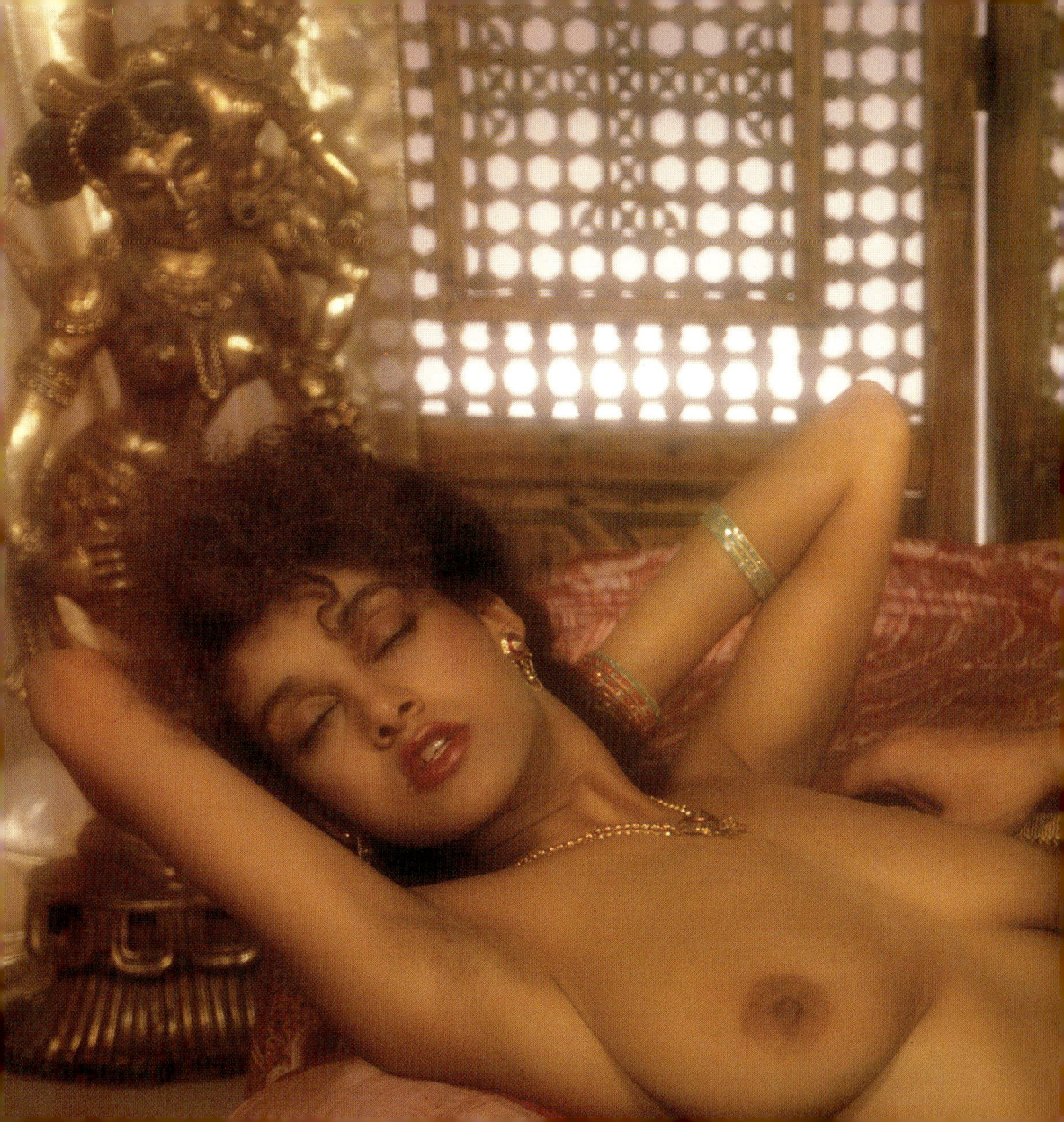

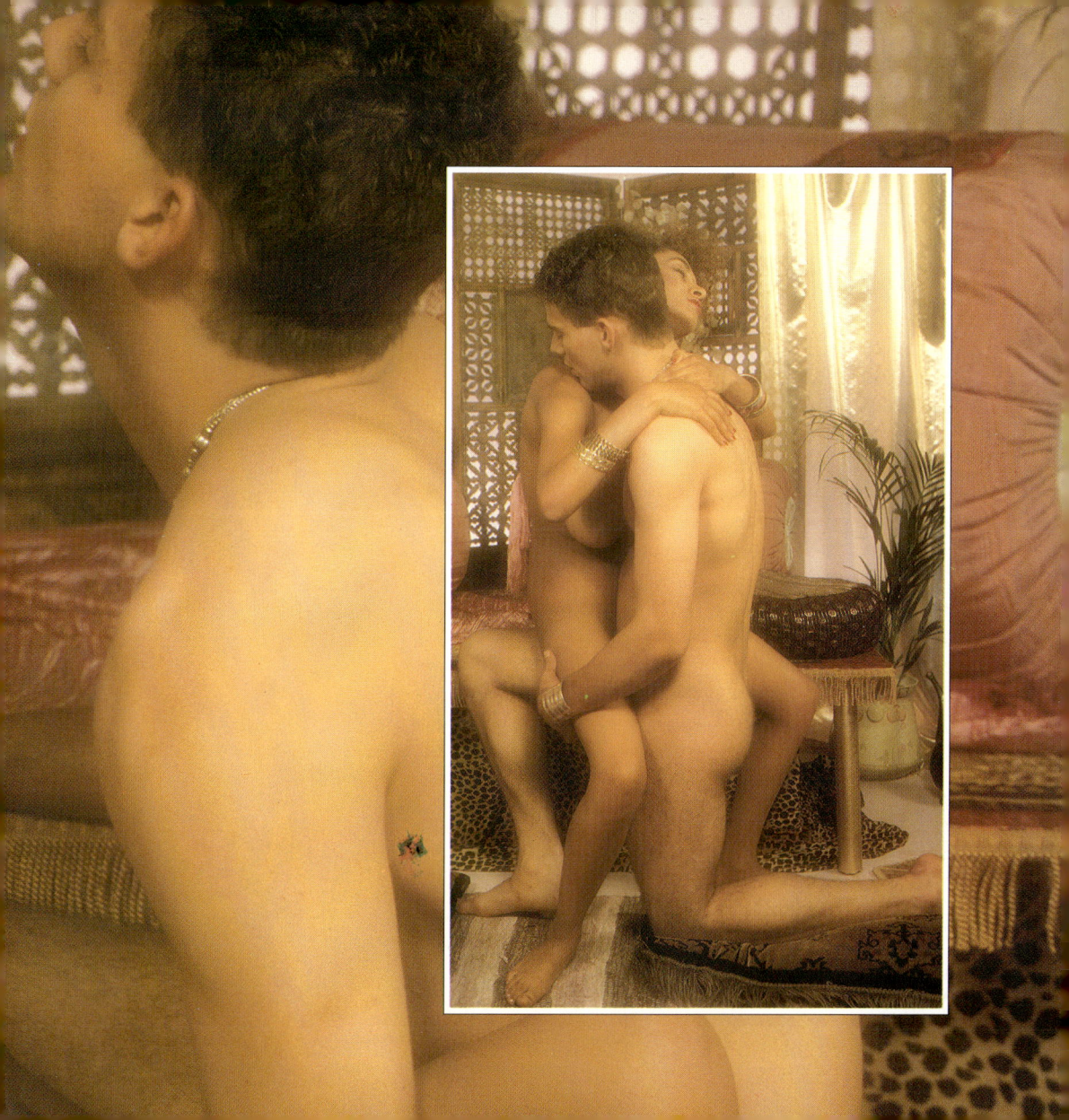

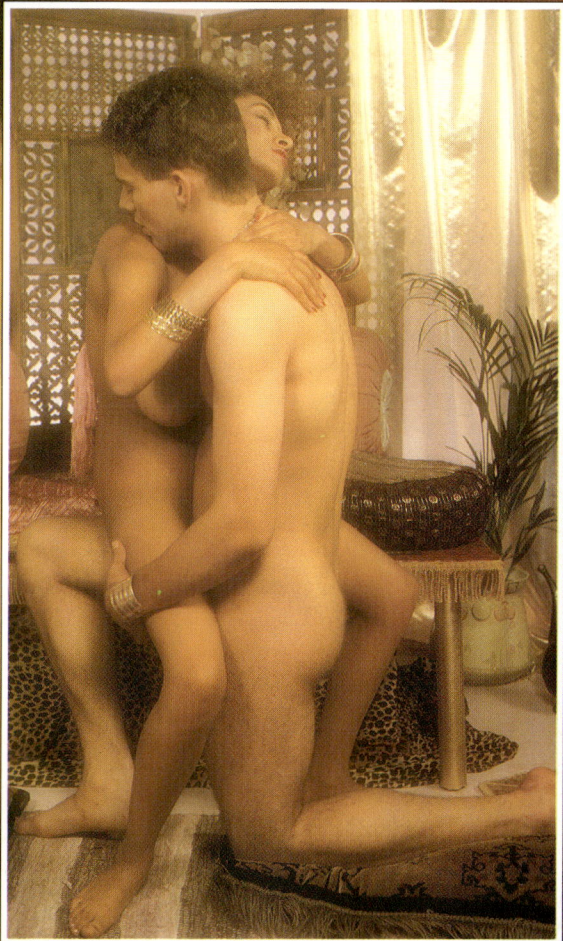

into the lingam could create an immediate and temporary effect if the user was psychologically conditioned to believe they would work.

The Kama Sutra warns that no aphrodisiac should be used which is doubtful in effect, which is likely to cause injury to the genitals, which involves deliberately killing animals and that involves the use of impure things. Users are advised to go to the experts for information and prescriptions - scientists, magicians and older, trusted relatives.

This section of recipes brings the book to an end, and the author makes it clear that the use of such things is something of a last resort. He would prefer that women and men gained the object of their desire through good looks, personality, knowledge and charm. And he would prefer that lovers were retained through an efficient but loving sexual technique.

The relevance of the Kama Sutra to readers today is more to do with attitude and spirit rather than to do with specific practices. We know much more about the way our bodies work today and have a much deeper insight into the ways in which desire can affect a person. But we also live in a much more complicated and tense society, so one of the messages of the book is to relax, take time to enjoy ourselves and each other and, above all, to seek knowledge about sex and treat it as a skill worth knowing about.

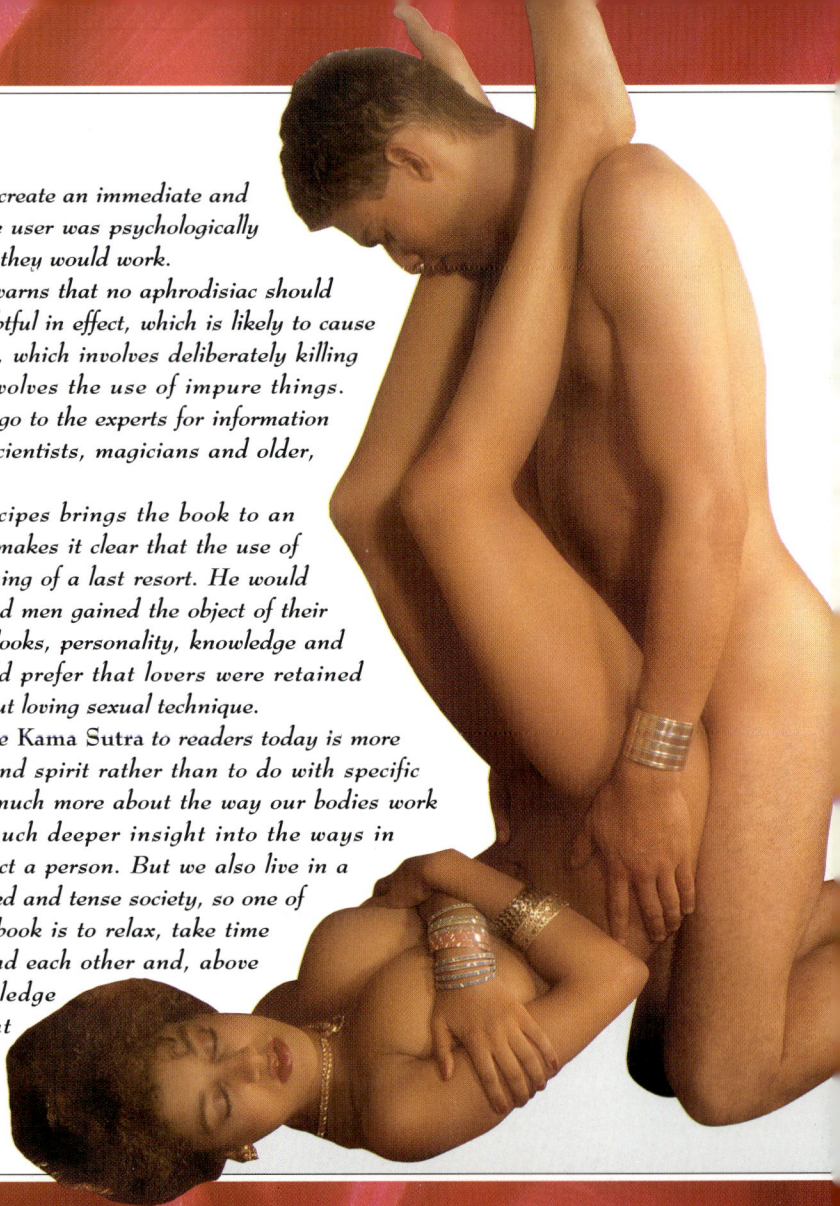

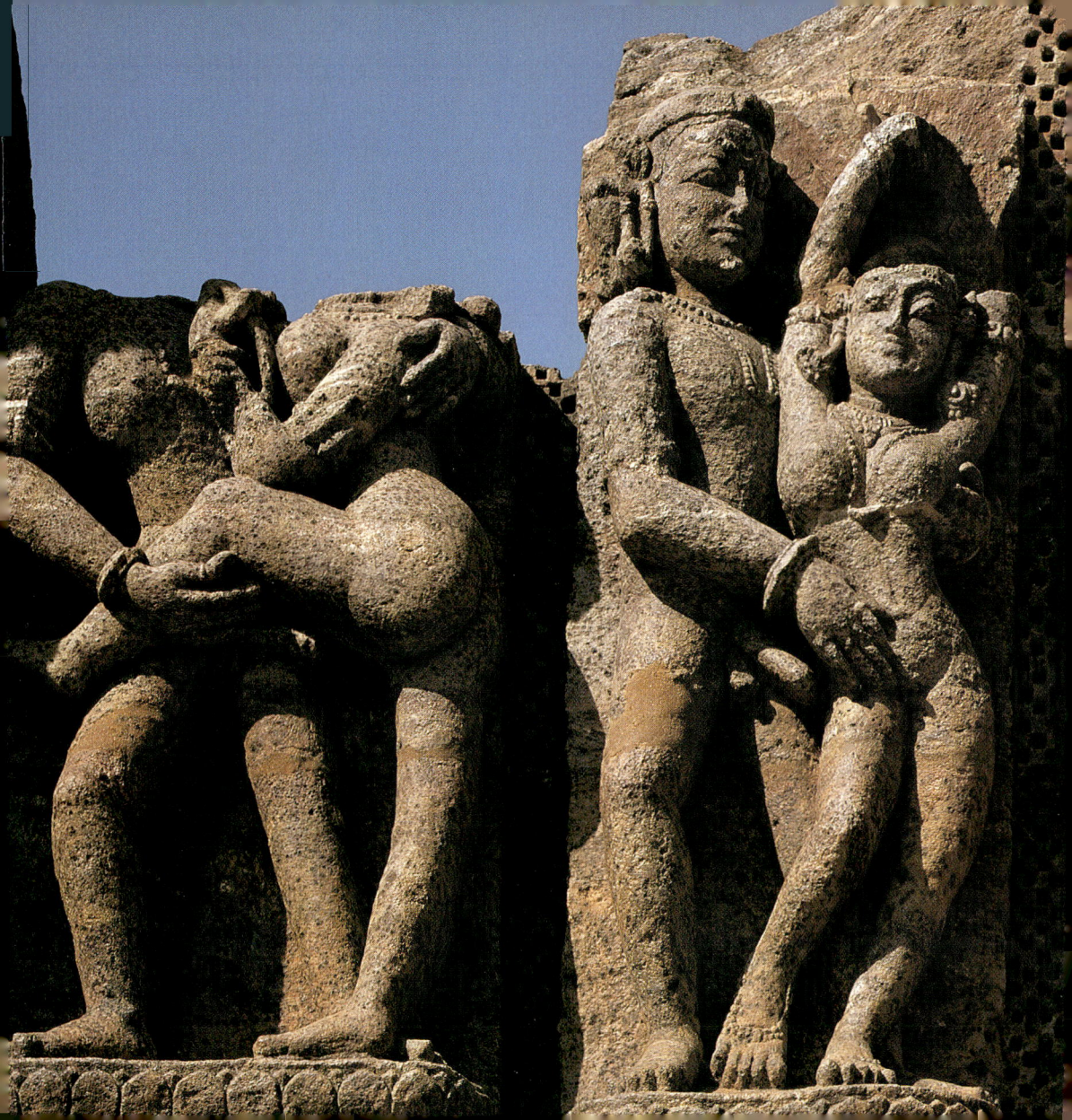

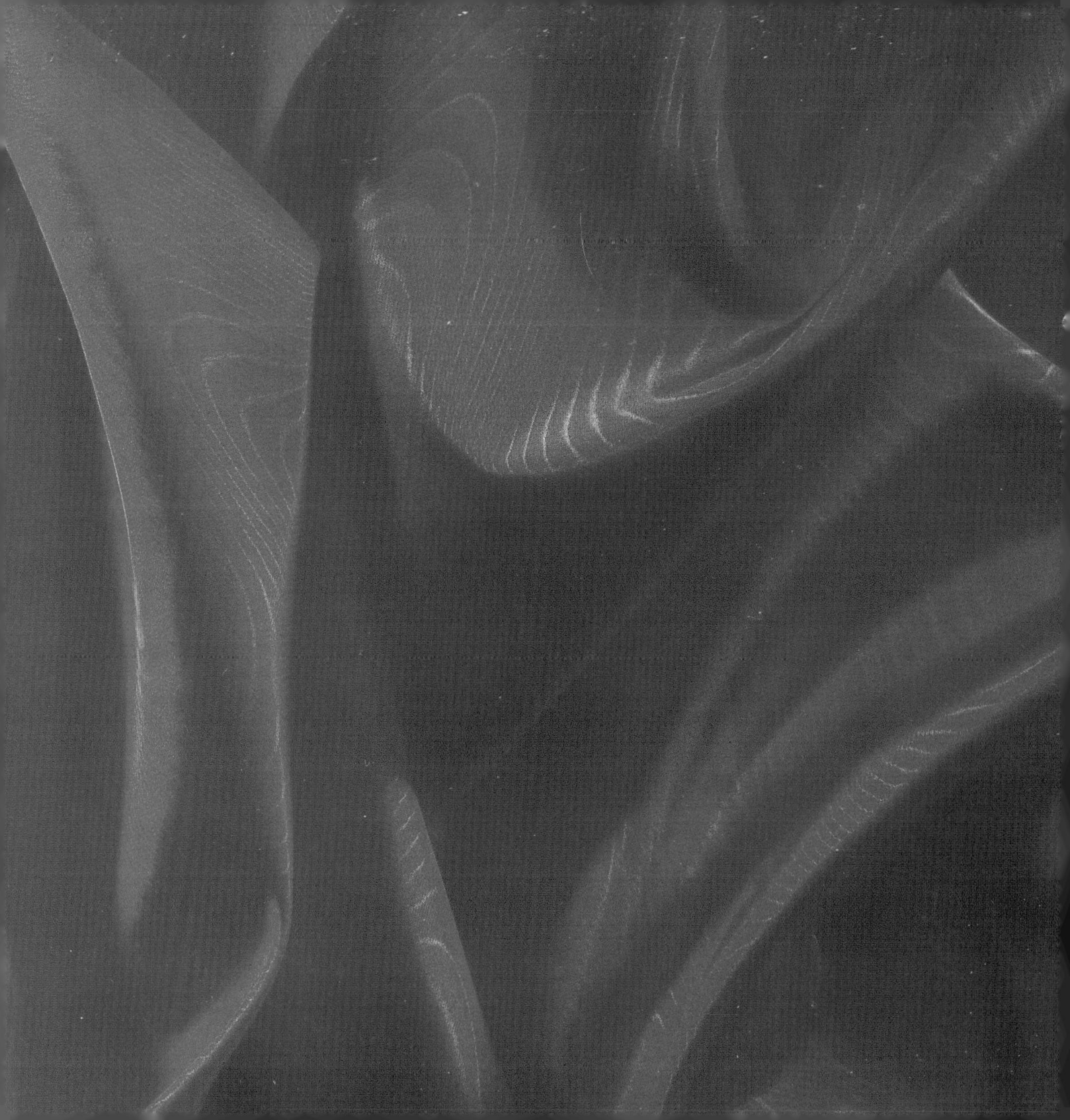